Translation, Disinformation

Michael Berry

Translation, Disinformation, and Wuhan Diary

Anatomy of a Transpacific Cyber Campaign

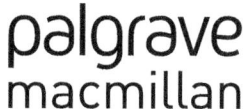

Michael Berry
Department of Asian Languages & Cultures
University of California, Los Angeles
LOS ANGELES, CA, USA

ISBN 978-3-031-16858-1   ISBN 978-3-031-16859-8   (eBook)
https://doi.org/10.1007/978-3-031-16859-8

Cover illustration © eStudio Calamar

This Palgrave Macmillan imprint is published by the registered company Springer Nature Switzerland AG.
The registered company address is: Gewerbestrasse 11, 6330 Cham, Switzerland

There is only one true test, and that is how you treat the weakest and most vulnerable members of your society.
—Fang Fang

for Fang Fang

Acknowledgments

The first draft of this book was written amid unusual circumstances; between June and November of 2020 I was still locked down at home in Los Angeles, California, requiring me to juggle between writing, online teaching, and constant supervision of my children whose elementary school classes had also migrated online due to COVID-19. Of course, there was also the ongoing disinformation campaign, which is the subject of this book, which was playing out in real time as I wrote. Special thanks to my wife Suk-Young Kim and my children, Miles and Naima, for their patience and support as I navigated the storm and did my best to document what was playing out. As I revised and expanded the manuscript throughout 2021 and into early 2022, I was fortunate to receive valuable feedback from David Der-wei Wang, Jing Tsu, Perry Link, Ian Johnson, John Nathan, Michael Emmerich, Ashley Esarey, Kaiser Kuo, and Jeffrey Wasserstrom. I want to single out my UCLA colleague King-Kok Cheung who not only provided strong moral support but also invaluable editorial input. The comments of the three external reviewers helped make this a better book. Between 2020 and 2022 I delivered several dozen (mostly online) lectures on *Wuhan Diary* and I benefited greatly from the comments and questions posed at all of those events, which provided me an opportunity to workshop some of the ideas presented in this book and prodded me to think about this project from new perspectives. Thanks to Liang Yanping, Wang Xiaoni, Erxiang, and all of those who supported Fang Fang, even in the face of threats and reprisals. Thanks to Alice Green, Cathy Scott, Sarah Hills, and Kiruthika Counassegarane at Palgrave

Macmillan for their support of this project, the editorial team at HarperVia, and Jennifer Lyons who championed this book from the beginning and has been an ardent supporter throughout this unusual journey. Final thanks go to Fang Fang, to whom I dedicate this book. May her model of bravery, tenacity, and commitment to truth continue to inspire and shine brightly.

CONTENTS

ABOUT THE AUTHOR

Michael Berry is Professor of Contemporary Chinese Cultural Studies at the University of California, Los Angeles (UCLA). Previously, he was Professor of Contemporary Chinese Cultural Studies and Director of the East Asia Center at the University of California, Santa Barbara. He holds a Ph.D. from Columbia University and his areas of research include modern and contemporary Chinese literature, Chinese cinema, popular culture in modern China, and translation studies.

Berry is the author of *A History of Pain: Trauma in Modern Chinese Literature and Film* (2008; 2017), which explores literary and cinematic representations of atrocity in twentieth-century China; *Speaking in Images: Interviews with Contemporary Chinese Filmmakers* (2005; 2006; 2007), a collection of dialogues with contemporary Chinese filmmakers including Hou Hsiao-hsien, Zhang Yimou, Stanley Kwan, and Jia Zhangke; the monograph, *Jia Zhang-ke's 'Hometown Trilogy': Xiao Wu, Platform, Unknown Pleasures* (2009; 2010), which offers extended analysis of the films *Xiao Wu, Platform*, and *Unknown Pleasures*; *Boiling the Sea: Hou Hsiao-hsien's Memories of Shadows and Light* (2014; 2015); *Jia Zhangke on Jia Zhangke* (2022); and *Enter the Clowns: The Queer Cinema of Cui Zi'en* (2022). He is also the editor of *The Musha Incident: A Reader on the Indigenous Uprising in Colonial Taiwan* (2022) and co-editor of *Modernism Revisited* (2016) and *Divided Lenses* (2016). He is also a contributor to numerous books and periodicals, including recent chapters in *The Oxford Handbook of Chinese Cinemas* (2013), *A Companion to Chinese*

Cinema (2012), *Electric Shadows: A Century of Chinese Cinema* (2014), *Columbia Companion to Modern Chinese Literature* (2016), *Harvard New Literary History of Modern China* (2016), and *The Chinese Cinema Book* (2018).

He is also the translator of several books, including *Hospital* (2023), *Wuhan Diary* (2020), *Remains of Life* (2017), *The Song of Everlasting Sorrow* (with Susan Chan Egan) (2008), *To Live* (2004), *Nanjing 1937: A Love Story* (2002), and *Wild Kids: Two Novels about Growing Up* (2000). His work has been recognized by two NEA Translation Grants (2008, 2021) and an Honorable Mention for the MLA Lois Roth Translation Prize (2009), and he has served on the jury for the Dream of the Red Chamber Prize (2012-2018) and on the jury member for numerous film festivals, including the Golden Horse Film Festival (2010, 2018).

LIST OF FIGURES

CHAPTER 1

Introduction: Origins

The first time I appeared in a Chinese newspaper was on May 21, 1994. As a foreign student living in Nanjing during that period, it wasn't uncommon to occasionally have some unusual visitors to our dormitory. Chinese students from nearby colleges would sometimes hang out in the lobby of our dorm hoping to strike up a conversation as a means of practicing their English; a philosophy professor once called on me, unannounced, and started lobbying for me to translate his new book *Nietzsche in China* (*Nicai zai Zhongguo* 尼采在中國)—it was the first time I had been invited to translate a book even though, at that time, I had only been studying Chinese for a few months—and on one occasion a friend brought a reporter from a local newspaper to my dorm room to meet me. The reporter didn't stay long and didn't say much; she certainly didn't mention that she was interested in writing a story about me. But, lo and behold, a few days later my name appeared in the pages of the *Fuwu daobao* 服務導報, or *Service Report*, a local Nanjing-based newspaper. The reporter had written an entire feature-length article on Chinese students who had foreign roommates in Nanjing entitled "What Foreigners Have Left Me With" ("Laowai gei wo liuxia le shenme?" 老外給我們留下了什麼?). The story featured an American college student by my name who was studying in Nanjing and was living in Xiyuan, my dorm at the time; but the rest of the details seemed peculiar. The story described how one night, just before my return to the United States, my Chinese roommate and I went up to the rooftop of our dormitory to recite poetry, gaze at the

© The Author(s), under exclusive license to Springer Nature Switzerland AG 2022
M. Berry, *Translation, Disinformation, and Wuhan Diary*, https://doi.org/10.1007/978-3-031-16859-8_1

moon, and embrace in tears. There was a homoerotic undercurrent running through the description but the truly queer thing about the story was the fact that I had not yet left China, I didn't have a Chinese roommate (which was generally not allowed in China at the time), and I did not have the habit of hanging out on the rooftop reciting classical Chinese love poems with my friends. Although this was more than 20 years before I would ever hear the term "fake news," I suppose that, in retrospect, this was the first time I was the subject of a fake news report. At the time, I was more amused than offended, but the experience did sew some seeds of caution when it came to how I viewed the media. If this harmless little story was the result of pure fabrication, what about the rest of what I was reading in the newspaper? I would have to wait another 25 years until I would get a taste of what happens when the full power of disinformation and "fake news" is truly unleashed.

One day when we look back upon the initial outbreak of COVID-19, we will all probably reflect upon where we were, how we were impacted, and what we did. In January of 2020, while many in the United States felt the coronavirus outbreak was still a world away, as a Chinese studies scholar it quickly began to sneak into my life. I started to follow the Chinese-language news coming out of Wuhan in January; many of my Chinese students, who were much more up to date on the latest coverage concerning the outbreak, began to wear face masks on campus; one colleague in my department adopted a "flexible attendance policy" (which the campus newspaper criticized as xenophobic at the time!); I witnessed some of my graduate students at UCLA spearhead a campaign to donate PPE to China; and, feeling I needed to do my part, I started reaching out to colleagues to organize a "teach-in" style event about the coronavirus.

On January 25, 2020, my old college friend, Simon, who works in IT for Disney, invited me and my kids to Disneyland for the day. I hesitated. Even at this early stage in the outbreak, we already knew about asymptomatic carriers and an incubation period that could be two weeks or longer. Knowing the virus was always several steps ahead of us, I carefully weighed whether or not to go. "Is this even safe?" But with zero confirmed cases in the Los Angeles area, I decided it should be okay. I texted Simon back on the morning of the 25th and told him that we were in. It did not take very long for me to regret my decision. It was the Chinese New Year and Disneyland had a special Spring Festival celebration; the park was overflowing with crowds of tourists, standing in long lines, eating fast-food version of Chinese cuisine like dumplings, steamed buns, and noodles, while watching Mickey Mouse and friends, decked out in bright, traditional-style Chinese clothing, perform Disney-fied versions of Lunar New Year dances. The very next day, January 26, 2020, Orange County, home to Disneyland, announced its first case of the novel coronavirus.

A few days after our trip to Disney, I began to get the feeling that something ominous was afoot. After reading more and more accounts about the Wuhan outbreak, I thought it would be a good idea to purchase some face masks and gloves. It was a Sunday night in late January when I decided it would be prudent to stock up on a few items. I told my wife I would make a quick trip to CVS and be back in a few minutes. I didn't expect the local CVS to be completely sold out. I drove to another CVS, and another, and another, and then a supermarket and a Walgreens. All of them were completely sold out of face masks; the only thing I was able to purchase was a single box of 50 latex surgical gloves. All other PPE was out of stock. As I went from store to store I could feel my desperation growing; it wouldn't be too much to say that I could feel a mild panic set in—not so much because I couldn't purchase any masks, but because it was the first time I was struck by the sense of how utterly unprepared we were for what was to come. At this point there was still only a small handful of confirmed coronavirus cases in Los Angeles and already there was a severe face mask shortage. I remember thinking, what are they going to do when there are 5000 cases? Or 50,000 cases?

On February 10, the event I had been working on, "The Novel Coronavirus: What Do We Know and What's Next?", one of the first "teach-in" style forums on the novel coronavirus was held. The forum, which I put together in conjunction with the UCLA Fielding School of Public Health, brought together scholars from a variety of disciplines including law, epidemiology, and infectious diseases in order to break down the latest knowledge he had about the virus. The topic of face masks actually came up, and, even though the infectious disease specialists assured the audience that masks were not needed, seeing 300 attendees packed together with not an empty seat in the room and only a small handful of people were wearing masks, I couldn't help but feel a bit concerned. There was a reception after the event where participants gathered around a table, nibbling on grapes and cookies; again, I wondered: "Is this even safe?" The following day, on February 11, 2020, the World Health Organization gave this novel coronavirus a new name: COVID-19.

I have always strived to find ways to make my teaching and research relevant outside of academia; sometimes that has taken the form of community outreach, media interface, or simply stressing practical applications in the classroom. When COVID-19 hit, the teach-in forum felt like a necessary response, but, deep down, I was struck by sense of helplessness. I was not an infectious disease specialist or a frontline worker, I never even took a CPR class; in the face of this existential threat, what could I possibly contribute?

Little did I know that, a few days earlier, as I had been navigating through the crowds of mouse-eared tourists at Disneyland with my six-year-old daughter, half a world away, in Wuhan, China, Fang Fang 方方 had just written the first entry of her diary. That was something I wouldn't learn about until later. But I did know Fang Fang, and, just a few months earlier, I had begun translating one of her novels. Fang Fang, one of China's most decorated writers, is actually the pen name for Wang Fang 汪芳, who was born in 1955 and was the former Chair of the Hubei Writers Association. Fang Fang began writing in the mid-1970s and has published more than 100 books, including novels, short stories, novellas, and essays. She has spent her entire life since the age of two in Wuhan, the country seat of Hubei province that is situated on the Yangtze and Han rivers. Many of Fang Fang's stories are set in Wuhan and she has authored numerous non-fiction accounts of the city, including the essay collections *The People of Wuhan* (*Wuhan ren* 武漢人) and *The Foreign Concessions of Hankou* (*Hankou zujie* 漢口租界). Often considered her masterpiece, the 1987 award-winning novella *The Scenery* (*Fengjing* 風景) has been considered a representative work of the neo-realist movement and been translated into numerous languages. In many ways, she is the single writer most often identified with the city Wuhan. So when the lockdown began in late January, Fang Fang seemed to be a natural candidate to chronicle what was happening.

I had been in periodic touch with Fang Fang regarding the translation of her novel *Soft Burial* (*Ruanmai* 軟埋). As the news coming out of Wuhan grew increasingly dire, I would occasionally reach out to her to make sure that she and her family were okay. We exchanged texts, but Fang Fang never even mentioned that she had started a blog, a quarantine, or lockdown diary (*fengcheng riji* 封城日記), as it had been referred to, about the coronavirus outbreak. I had noticed some posts on Weibo from Fang Fang about the situation in Wuhan, but had not read them in detail. It wasn't until after a phone call with my colleague and former doctoral advisor David Der-wei Wang, who suggested I take a closer look at the diary, that I finally sat down to read some of her entries.

That was in early February, Wuhan was more than a week into their lockdown and Fang Fang had already posted several diary entries online. Beginning on January 25, Fang Fang would post her entries late at night, usually between 11:00 PM and 3:00 am, recording her experience under quarantine. *Wuhan Diary* became one of the most important chronicles of the COVID-19 outbreak in Wuhan and rapidly generated a loyal following of tens of millions of readers (before it would ultimately become the target of an online smear campaign and end up being washed from the internet). I read one or two entries and was immediately struck by the immediacy and power of Fang Fang's message. I had been following the official news reports coming out of Wuhan, but nothing I had read was able to put a human face on the crisis the way Fang Fang's diary did. And nothing I had read conveyed the devastating impact of the coronavirus like Fang Fang's accounts. Over the course of my career I had translated several books, mostly contemporary Chinese novels, and I had always carefully read each work cover-to-cover to decide if I wanted to invest the time to translate the work. Never before had I made a decision to translate a book based on just a few chapters, let alone a book that was still being written. In all fairness, at the time, *Wuhan Diary* was not even a book, just a handful of blog entries that had gone viral on the Chinese internet. But I was immediately swept away by the power and immediacy of Fang Fang's writing. It was no wonder that, virtually overnight, Fang Fang had become a hero to millions of netizens in China during the early days of the Wuhan lockdown. I made a snap decision. On February 16 I texted Fang Fang suggesting we temporarily table *Soft Burial* and I instead begin translating her diary.

But Fang Fang hesitated. She thanked me for my interest in the diary but cautioned, "The coronavirus outbreak is still ongoing, I'm also still writing my diary. So at the moment I don't have any publication plans. If you don't mind, let's wait until after this outbreak has passed, okay?" While I remained firmly convinced that what Fang Fang was writing was of great importance, I naturally respected her wishes. A week later, on February 24, after other overseas publishers and media outlets began to reach out to Fang Fang, she got back in touch with me and agreed to collaborate. I immediately pushed my other book projects aside and the following day began translating what would eventually become *Wuhan Diary* (*Wuhan riji* 武漢日記). I toiled around the clock, working harder on this project than any other book in my career—the virus was spreading, the clock was ticking, and the world needed to hear Fang Fang's voice.

I was exactly one month behind Fang Fang when I began translating, and, as fast as I worked—translating approximately **5000** words a day, seven days a week, for just over a month—it still felt like I wasn't fast enough; day after day, there were news reports about new COVID-19 hot spots all over the world. Just two weeks after beginning my translation, Los Angeles fell under lockdown, and, by the time the English edition of *Wuhan Diary* was published in mid-May, the United States was already firmly in the clutches of the novel coronavirus. All of the things that Fang Fang described in her diary—which in February and March felt like messages from a strange dystopian future—were now part of our everyday reality. Unfortunately, many of the lessons in Fang Fang's diary that Chinese readers had learned early would take a lot longer for residents of the United States to learn. Even as COVID-19 spread across Europe and the United States, many in the West still resisted face masks, social distancing, and lockdown protocols. Having vicariously experienced the Wuhan lockdown through Fang Fang's eyes, I was well aware of the devastating impact the novel coronavirus unleashed upon a city that *did implement* the strictest quarantine measures; I dreaded what would become of the United States as they failed to heed the warnings. People were not wearing face masks; there was no federal strategy implemented for testing, tracking, and tracing; and the US government response to COVID-19 had unthinkably been transformed into a "political issue." It was as if Wuhan never happened and the lessons Fang Fang had shared were all in vain. In some sense, I felt as if I failed.

All the while, a complex set of forces began to align that transformed *Wuhan Diary* into something much more than just a book; it became a cultural phenomenon. Ding Fan 丁帆 described the unprecedented manner in which the diary captured the collective imagination of people all over China:

> For the past century, a widespread enlightened consciousness has never once touched so many people so deeply, at least without it being forced or compulsory; 50 million people staying up past midnight each night just wanting to read the next installment of Fang Fang's diary—the scene of all those people reading is shocking to imagine and it singlehandedly broke through the traditional limits of literature.[1]

[1] Feng Yunkan. "Check Out Which Specialists Support Fang Fang and Who is Against Her" ("Kankan zhichi he fandui Fang Fang de zhuanjia dou you shei?" 看看支持和反對方方的專家都有誰?) https://zhuanlan.zhihu.com/p/133760882

But as the diary became headline news and Fang Fang became a veritable celebrity in the Chinese speaking community and, eventually, around the world, a darker set of forces also began to coalesce around her account. The diary became the subject of political cartoons, heated debates among Chinese public intellectuals, the target of rap-style diss songs, and hordes of internet trolls who launched a protracted media campaign against the book. Eventually, I too got pulled into the attacks. "Stupid dog!", "Go Fuck yourself, shame on u," "How does the steamed bun soaked in human blood taste? You white skinned pig!" Those are just three of the messages I received on April 8 on my Weibo account. Seemingly overnight, my Weibo message board was flooded by thousands of aggressive, explicative-laden messages and threats. As the attacks began to surge, I began to feel increasingly self-conscious about how my work was being appropriated by different political forces; as uncomfortable as I felt about being demonized by ultra-nationalist forces in China, I felt equally squeamish when media outlets abroad (such as a Falun Gong-run television station) ran stories about the attacks I was receiving through a highly anti-China lens. A few weeks after the attacks were launched I also began to receive a wellspring of letters of support and solidarity from Chinese readers who were appalled by the way I had been targeted. I suddenly found myself amid an increasingly complex, politicized, and polarized ideological tug of war. At the same time, I knew that what I was experiencing was but a small taste of what Fang Fang was going through in China. But what was at stake went far beyond *Wuhan Diary;* it was a story that involved translation, COVID-19, the US-China trade war, cyber-politics, disinformation campaigns, and the role of writing as testimony, civil engagement, and community building.

While the events unfolding in China around *Wuhan Diary* (and the larger thrust to control political narratives surrounding COVID-19) were a unique case study and I am by no means attempting to argue for an equivalency, there are important parallels to be drawn. As I personally drew lessons from the "Fang Fang Incident" about the current state of culture and politics in China, so too I was seeing warped reflections of those same lessons playing out in headline news around the world as the pandemic spread. Many of those lessons were particularly prescient when it came to a set of similar dynamics simultaneously unfolding in the United States. These parallels demonstrated just how powerful the lessons of *Wuhan Diary* had been in not only capturing the zeitgeist of the early-COVID-19 era in China, but also in projecting and predicting so many of the more disturbing global trends of the pandemic—an uptick in authoritarianism, misinformation, and political extremism. Whereas Donald Trump praised Xi Jinping for his response early on, he quickly revised his stance when COVID-19 reached US shores. Members of the Trump administration began to racialize the virus not only by using disparaging terms like "China Virus," "Wuhan Virus," and "Kung Flu," but also repeatedly blaming the entire pandemic on the Chinese Communist Party and threatening payback. But as each side pointed fingers, setting in motion an "othering process" whereby the other side is framed as an adversary, what we actually see is a mirroring effect. Caught in a cycle of mutual provocation, each side took increasingly aggressive punitive actions against the other, leading to a cycle of continued escalation. The story of what happened to *Wuhan Diary* was therefore very much caught up in a transpacific ideological tug of war that played out not just on Weibo, WeChat, and the *Global Times*, but also on Facebook, Twitter, and Fox News.

This is a book that attempts to navigate a series of disparate yet interwoven questions through the lens of a single book; it is, in some sense, a tale of two viruses. In one of the very first book-length publications on COVID-19, *Pandemic!: COVID-19 Shakes the World*, Slavoj Žižek had already begun to pinpoint the intersection between these two viral contagions when he wrote:

> The ongoing spread of the coronavirus epidemic has also triggered a vast epidemic of ideological viruses which were lying dormant in our societies: fake news, paranoiac conspiracy theories, explosions of racism. The well-grounded medical need for quarantines found an echo in the ideological pressure to establish clear borders and to quarantine enemies who pose a threat to our identity.[2]

But through this unique case study of *Wuhan Diary*, we are offered a rare glimpse into not only the anatomy and evolution of a COVID-19 narrative, but also the viral debates about Chinese civil society and the role of the disinformation campaigns that evolved alongside it. It is an attempt to home in on one specific campaign that began to play out in March 2020, running parallel with the global spread of COVID-19, twisting,

[2] Zizek, Slavoj. *Pandemic!: COVID-19 Shakes the World*. New York: Polity Press, 2020. Pg. 39.

expanding, going viral, and mutating in the many months to follow. As it evolved, a narrative about the lockdown in Wuhan would get pulled into a myriad of parallel controversies, repeatedly reinforcing Žižek's claim that "viral infections work hand in hand in both dimensions: real and virtual."[3] As the translator of *Wuhan Diary*, this is an odd book for me to write. As an author, most of my books have had more critical distance; in this case, not only were the events playing out as I was writing about them, but I also played a direct role in the story that was unfolding. This provided me with a unique vantage point from which to understand how the controversy evolved and also made me privy to details to which very few others had access to. In that sense, this book vacillates between a highly personal narrative and a more distanced discussion and analysis of what was playing out.

Initially I had no plans to write a book like this. Having just spent several months living, breathing, and sleeping *Wuhan Diary*, I was eager to get back to other long-overdue book projects, but this was a book I had to write. The more attacks I received and the more articles about *Wuhan Diary* that I noticed "disappearing" from the internet only increased my drive to document what was happening: to bear testimony to what I have witnessed and experienced. I'm sure that many of my detractors will read this short book as an attempt to "vilify" China; it is not. It is an attempt to provide a nuanced understanding of the complex set of political and cultural circumstances that played out around a translation project that I was intimately involved with. The controversy surrounding *Wuhan Diary* evolved so quickly and unexpectedly that, as I was racing to translate the book, it often felt like the very ground beneath my feet was shifting.

In some sense, this book also serves as a rejoinder to months of consistent attacks and online harassment. When the online attacks initially broke out there was a strong urge to respond forcefully in real time; however, given the tactics being employed (a machinegun-like barrage of lies and disinformation), death threats meant to intimidate, not to mention the sheer number of attacks being waged, it quickly became clear that a different approach would be needed. Posting counter-arguments on Weibo would be akin to getting down in the mud and wrestling with the trolls. I instead chose to respond through more official channels: a translator's afterword to *Wuhan Diary* in order to better contextualize the book, an op-ed with *The Washington Post* to break down how a translator of a diary

---

[3] Ibid. Pg. 44.

could be targeted with online threats and attacks, interviews with reputable new outlets, and now this book. At the same time, over the course of writing this book I have been keenly aware of the unusual factors that contributed to its writing. Part of those circumstances have perhaps contributed to the book's sometimes defensive tone. That is not by accident. After seeing and experiencing how *Wuhan Diary*, the author, and myself were subjected to slander, lies, and brutal attacks, this became a way to set the record straight and provide an accurate record of what really transpired. Part of that also impacted the very structure of this book. For instance, I would have never normally thought to devote an entire chapter to how the title of a translated book was conceived. Even the thought of such an exercise feels self-absorbed (and not likely very compelling to your average reader), but when the very title of a book elicits thousands of attacks based upon groundless suppositions and lies, as was the case with *Wuhan Diary*, a full contextualization was called for.

I also see this book as a gesture of preservation. As I was translating *Wuhan Diary* I was continually haunted by the shadow of disappearance. Not only were many of Fang Fang's diary entries deleted from the internet in China, but hundreds of articles and posts about the diary were also erased without a trace. Initially it was only pro-Fang Fang posts that were being deleted; however, by August 2020 I started to notice that even some of the anti-Fang Fang posts, including an entire e-book aimed at discrediting the diary that had been uploaded to Amazon.com under the title *Great Wuhan But Bad Diary*, had completely disappeared. As I saw pieces of the digital footprint left in the wake of *Wuhan Diary* being systematically dismantled and erased, the urge, if not responsibility, to document this story felt all the more pressing. And so I began to document all of the stories, letters, tweets, texts, messages, and posts that had been collectively constructing the story behind *Wuhan Diary* and the so-called Fang Fang Incident.

There is no way any one person can ever truly understand all of the complex and twisted machinations that transpired behind the scenes and all of the nuanced views that so many disparate groups of Chinese netizens held about the controversy—there were simply too many voices involved, from legal scholars to linguists, from specialists in discourse analysis to advocates for human rights and, of course, the thousands of online trolls. I don't think there can ever be a definitive account of what happened during the first several months of 2020 when *Wuhan Diary* took China by storm, but this is my attempt to make sense of it for myself and for those readers who want to understand how a diary could elicit one of the most heated intellectual, political, and societal debates to be carried out in decades about a book. The controversy was so intense that, in many ways, it seemed reminiscent of the attacks waged against Katherine Mayo's *Mother India* in 1927 or Salman Rushdie's *The Satanic Verses* in 1989. In the case of Mayo's polemical attack on Indian independence, "numerous public protest meetings were held against the book in various parts of the world" and "few books have ever come close to matching *Mother India* in provoking fury and such vehement support across several continents."[4] Rushdie's *The Satanic Verses* triggered attacks, denunciations, calls to ban the book, death threats, and even the murder of the book's Japanese translator.[5] For *The Satanic Verses*, these attacks were inspired by extremist religious views, but in the case of *Wuhan Diary* it was extremist nationalistic views fueling the fire. What was truly unique about the attacks against *Wuhan* Diary, however, was the way in which online discourse had been manipulated, pivoting overnight from widespread support to mass denunciation. Of course, the final word on *Wuhan Diary* has yet to be written and its afterlife continues to evolve. After facing widespread denunciations and attacks and being largely erased from online discourse, Fang Fang's *Wuhan Diary* returned to public discourse in China in January 2022 during the Xi'an lockdown and again in April 2022 during the citywide lockdown of Shanghai. Suddenly netizens began calling out how "Xi'an needs a Fang Fang" and "Shanghai needs its own Fang Fang"; one woman from Shanghai who publicly attacked Fang Fang in 2020 publicly apologized to her after her own city came under lockdown.

[4] Sinha Mrinalini. *Specters of Mother India: The Global Restructuring of an Empire*. Durham: Duke University Press, 2006. Pg. 2.

[5] In the case of *The Satanic Verses*, the denunciation of the book led to numerous deaths, injuries, and assassination attempts. The book's Japanese translator, Hitoshi Igarashi (1947–1991), was tragically murdered in response to the issuing of fatwas calling for the death of the author "and of those involved in its publication who are aware of its content." Other individuals targeted included the book's Italian translator Ettore Capriolo, who was stabbed multiple times; William Nygaard, the book's Norwegian publisher, who suffered from multiple gunshot wounds after a failed assassination attempt; and Aziz Nesin, the book's Turkish translator, who was targeted in an attack which led to the death of 37 people, while Nesin escaped. Then on August 12, 2022 the author himself was the victim of an attempted murder while preparing to deliver a public lecture in Chautauqua, New York. While there were no deaths or physical injuries associated with the campaign against *Wuhan Diary*, there was an abundance of hate speech, death threats, and a mass "hate campaign" carried out online that echoed a similar intolerance as seen in the attacks against Rushdie's book.

Understanding this storm of controversy is not just about understanding contemporary China, for me it was also very much about understanding the United States. Besides serving as a window through which to examine the origins, intentions, and functions of a mass disinformation campaign, this book also serves as a mirror for how similar campaigns play out at home. The deeper I became drawn into the storm surrounding *Wuhan Diary*, the more keenly I became aware of the fact that all of the things I saw playing out around the book—online attacks by bots and trolls, conspiracy theories, lapses in government accountability, the rise of "fake news," attempts to suppress books, control of social media, the breakdown of civil discourse and deep fissures in the very fabric of civil society—were also making headline news every day in Trump's America. Somehow *Wuhan Diary* and the controversy surrounding its publication captured the zeitgeist of the moment; at times it felt as if the book was a microcosm, or even a metaphor, for the age we were living in. But *Wuhan Diary* is not a metaphor: the stakes were very real, and this is the story of how one woman's pandemic diary would capture the hearts of tens of millions of readers before going on to spark a nationwide debate that would test the limits of civil discourse in Chinese society and divide a nation.

CHAPTER 2

Viral Diary

When Fang Fang uploaded her first diary entry on January 25, 2020, it was something of an experiment. It was a short post of only 433 Chinese characters (it would be the shortest entry in the entire 60-day chronicle) and described how the editor of the influential Chinese literary journal *Harvest* (*Shouhuo* 收穫), Cheng Yongxin 程永新, had reached out in hopes of her writing a series of essays on the outbreak. In some ways, Fang Fang's description is reminiscent of Lu Xun's 魯迅 "Preface to *A Call to Arms*" (*Na han zixu* 呐喊自序) written almost exactly a hundred years earlier in 1922. In his "Preface," an iconic document that would provide an "origin story" for the birth of modern Chinese literature, Lu Xun recalled how he was commissioned to contribute to the literary journal *New Youth* (*Xin qingnian* 新青年) by its editor, Chen Duxiu 陳獨秀. Lu Xun hesitated. He questioned the efficacy of literature as a tool to "wake people up" and used the metaphor of the iron house to highlight his point:

> "Imagine an iron house without windows, absolutely indestructible, with many people fast asleep inside who will soon die of suffocation. But you know since they will die in their sleep, they will not feel the pain of death. Now if you cry aloud to wake a few of the lighter sleepers, making those unfortunate few suffer the agony of irrevocable death, do you think you are doing them a good turn?"
>
> "But if a few awake, you can't say there is no hope of destroying the iron house."

M. Berry, *Translation, Disinformation, and Wuhan Diary*, https://doi.org/10.1007/978-3-031-16859-8_2

True, in spite of my own conviction, I could not blot out hope, for hope lies in the future. I could not use my own evidence to refute his assertion that it might exist.[1]

Lu Xun would of course put his reservations aside and contribute to *New Youth*, and the 1918 short story he published there "A Madman's Diary" (Kuangren riji 狂人日記) would go on to be regarded as one of the first truly "modern" works of Chinese fiction. Partially inspired by Gogol's work of the same name, "A Madman's Diary" attempted to expose the visible and invisible structures of violence and cannibalism, both literal and metaphoric, woven into the fabric of society. The diary was a purely fictional story, but through that lens of fictionality, Lu Xun's story would reveal deep truths about the society in which he lived. "A Madman's Diary" would also spark new discussions and debates about history, ethics, language, and the very nature of the Chinese national character and civil society. With one foot in tradition and one foot in modernity, it was a period of transition for China: "A Diary of Madman" tapped into the inner struggle and tortured soul of a nation (and a writer) in inner-revolt, in the process of becoming.

A century later, when Fang Fang responded to Cheng Yongxin's invitation, she also hesitated. Fang Fang's reluctance, however, seemed to be less rooted in reservations about the power of literature to impact society—unlike Lu Xun, who was at the beginning of his career as a fiction writer, Fang Fang had already spent more than four decades as a professional writer in China—she instead worried about something seemingly more mundane: "will [the diary] even be able to be posted."[2] For the vast majority of her career, Fang Fang has enjoyed a prestigious position in Chinese literary circles; however, she was now finding it increasingly difficult to enjoy unencumbered access to social media. After having several earlier posts deleted from her preferred social media platform of Sina Weibo, Fang Fang was unsure if her new posts would even be able to be successfully uploaded. She even asked her readers to leave a comment in the thread below her post to let her know if that first entry was successfully uploaded or not. It seemed like a minor detail at the time, but the reference to online censorship, the uncertainty regarding the role of

[1] Lu Hsun. *Selected Stories*. New York: W.W. Norton, 2003. Pg. 5.
[2] Fang Fang. *Wuhan Diary: Dispatches from a Quarantined City*. New York: HarperVia, 2020. Pg. 4.

technology and its "reliability" in transmitting stories, and the realization "that technology can sometimes be every bit as evil as a contagious virus"[3] would also prove prophetic as *Wuhan Diary* went on to find itself embroiled in a complex web of cyber-politics. Whereas Lu Xun's "A Madman's Diary" was fiction that revealed inner societal and cultural truths, *Wuhan Diary* was a factual account that would be accused of harboring "fictions"; while Lu Xun's diary revealed the shocking underbelly of cultural cannibalism lurking beneath the surface of society, the response to Fang Fang's diary unveiled a destructive, viral contagion threatening to create even greater rifts in online discourse and society at large; where Lu Xun's story launched a literary revolution, Fang Fang's diary would set in motion one of the most heated and explosive literary and political debates in contemporary China.

Of course on the surface, Fang Fang's diary accounts on the novel coronavirus outbreak in Wuhan during early 2020 are a world away from Lu Xun's fictional diary from 1918. *Wuhan Diary* vacillates between mundane everyday details (like what to do when you run out of dog food and all the pet stores are closed), passages where the author relays medical information about transmission and the severity of the virus (including DIY prevention tips like taking hot showers, loading up with vitamin C, and drinking a lot of hot water), updates from medical professionals about the overall outbreak situation in Wuhan, information passed down from news articles and videos the author has seen, advice for fellow residents on cooperating with lockdown ordinances, and regular updates about how she and her friends, colleagues, and family members were weathering the crisis. And then there were poetic passages that deeply affected millions of readers. "*When an era sheds a speck of dust it might not seem like much, but when it falls upon the shoulders of an individual it feels like a mountain*" was a line from the diary that took on a life its own: it was quoted, forwarded, and shared by countless readers, capturing the fear, uncertainty, and random nature of the way the virus struck, and eventually it became the first desolate anthem of the COVID-19 era. Fang Fang also used her public platform to raise awareness about subjects seldom talked about in mainstream Chinese society; for instance, there are numerous passages where she openly discusses the psychological toll of the lockdown, anticipating the dire need for psychological counseling and support. This itself proved

---

[3] Ibid.

to be an important intervention considering how guarded and shunned open discussions of mental health issues are in China.[4]

Over the course of the diary, there were also a series of incredible passages where Fang Fang expressed her frustration and anger with early missteps, including the disorganized response during the initial outbreak, the attempt to silence early whistleblowers like Dr. Li Wenliang 李文亮, and incidents where she felt politics were placed above public health. With these passages, there were also calls for officials to assume "responsibility" by apologizing to the public and resigning in cases where their actions contributed to human losses. For those outside of Hubei province, *Wuhan Diary* became a portal to understand what was occurring there, and, for those living in Wuhan, the diary provided comfort so that, as millions of residents quarantined inside their homes, they knew they were never alone. In the eyes of many, Fang Fang became a keeper of memory. In the words of award-winning novelist Yan Lianke 閻連科, who early on spoke out in support of the diary:

> Imagine this: the author Fang Fang did not exist in today's Wuhan. She did not keep records or pen down her personal memories and feelings. Neither were there tens of thousands of people who were like Fang Fang and would send out loud cries for help via their mobile phone. What would we have heard? What would we have seen?[5]

Yan Lianke's rhetorical questions point to just how vitally important Fang Fang's testimony was to so many readers. Throughout the coronavirus outbreak, Fang Fang continued to document not only what was happening on the ground through the sharing of personal stories from her friends, family, and neighbors, but she also provided a fascinating glimpse into how Chinese internet culture was reacting to the outbreak. As the coronavirus spread and people were desperate for not just information, but also human connection, so too Fang Fang's diary "went viral," shared online by over 50 million people in China. More than anyone else, Fang Fang

---

[4] For more on the intersection of mental health issues and the pandemic in China, see Vivian Wang and Javier C. Hernandez. "China Long Avoided Discussing Mental Health. The Pandemic Changed That." New York Times, December 21, 2020. https://www.nytimes.com/2020/12/21/world/asia/china-covid-mental-health.html.

[5] Yan Lianke. "What Happens After Coronavirus? On Community Memory and Repeating Our Own Mistakes" March 11, 2020 on Literary Hub. https://lithub.com/yan-lianke-what-happens-after-coronavirus/

emerged as *the voice* for Wuhan; and her diary became a place for Chinese readers to visit for solace, comfort, an emotional release, to learn about the latest developments concerning the outbreak, and, sometimes, just to "check in" on the author.

As the diary unfolded, there were also marked shifts in tone and focus as Fang Fang wrote. During the first two thirds or so of the diary, as existential questions weighed heavy, more of the diary focused upon documenting a complex and ever-evolving situation. There was a consistent emphasis on the number of new patients infected with COVID-19, the status of available beds at major hospitals, and an urgent set of pleas that coronavirus patients get proper treatment and patients suffering from other existing ailments not get overlooked in the process. However, as hospitals acquired the needed PPE, an influx of medical workers came into Wuhan to provide additional support, and the overall number of patients began to decline, the tone of *Wuhan Diary* began to transform. Fang Fang began to spend more time reflecting upon the aforementioned topic of "accountability" (*zhuize* 追責/*wenze* 問責). As those calls for accountability increased in frequency, so too did the frequency of the online attacks against Fang Fang. Eventually, these cyber-attacks, discussions of online censorship, and direct engagement with online trolls became an increasingly important sub-theme of the diary itself. As her diary began to take on more complex questions related to online attacks and troll culture, Fang Fang's entries also dramatically increased in length. Where early entries tally around 1214 characters (January 27) to around 1660 (January 29), later entries roughly double in length, such as 3034 characters (March 17) or 3229 characters (March 18). Most importantly, over the course of those final entries, the tone of the diary also transformed; as Professor Wang Jiaxin 王家新 from Renmin University noted: "Fang Fang persisted with her writing not only as she was under attack but even when she was facing personal threats to her safety. And not only did she continue writing, but she became even more 'fierce' as she went. Almost every installment of her diary would commit another great violation.[…] This diary is no simple personal record, it is a voice speaking out against violence and lies."[6] The "ferocity" that Fang Fang harnessed in the latter portions of her diary was a characteristic that would prove alternately refreshingly

---

[6] Feng Yukan. "Check Out Which Specialists Support Fang Fang and Who is Against Her" ("Kankan zhichi he fandui Fang Fang de zhuanjia dou you shei? 看看支持和反對方方的專家都有誰?) https://zhuanlan.zhihu.com/p/133760882

inspiring for those who saw in her a voice speaking out against injustice and maddingly threatening to those who viewed her words as transgressive and potentially destabilizing.

There are many narrative threads running through *Wuhan Diary*, making it a complex text, a pastiche of interwoven thoughts, themes, and responses. Fedtke, Ibahrine, and Wang have described the diary from the perspectives of sousveillance and solidarity: "sousveillance as the guiding principle in Fang Fang's work to guarantee accountability of responsible officials" and "solidarity as a means to contain the pandemic and misinfodemic."[7] But even within the framework of sousveillance, Fang Fang's diary undergoes a shift. Early on, *Wuhan Diary* could be considered very closely aligned with "in-band sousveillance" (especially given Fang Fang's standing with official government organizations like the Hubei Writers Association); however, as the diary gradually took on a more critical tone, it became more closely aligned to out-of-band sousveillance, which is unwelcome by the organization.[8] There was also a collective facet to the diary, which as Kevin Robins has pointed out:

> ...through the great montage of diverse, competing, and frequently clashing accounts, what Fang Fang manages to pull together, in my view, is precisely a kind of *Wirgeschichte* [we-story], a collective telling of multitudinous lives and their collective entanglements.[9]

While highly personal, the diary also drew from countless sources and perspectives, indeed wielding a collective power. Eventually the two primary narrative strains that emerge from the diary concern the coronavirus outbreak and the online attacks. These dual narratives, while superficially seem to be of two different worlds, actually run parallel: they feed one another and speak to different strains of virality. Their intertwined existence also helps explain how a diary could go on to spark a nationwide

---

[7] Fedtke, Jana, Mohammed Ibahrine, and Yuting Wang. "Corona crisis chronicle: Fang Fang's *Wuhan Diary* (2020) as an act of sousveillance" *Online Information Review* February 23, 2021. Pg. 800. https://www.emerald.com/insight/1468-4527.htm

[8] These comments are drawn partially from interview statements given to Fedtke, Ibahrine, and Wang and quoted in their article: Fedtke, Jana, Mohammed Ibahrine, and Yuting Wang. "Corona crisis chronicle: Fang Fang's *Wuhan Diary* (2020) as an act of sousveillance" *Online Information Review* February 23, 2021. Pg. 804. https://www.emerald.com/insight/1468-4527.htm.

[9] Kevin Robins. "The Great City is Fragile: Fang Fang's *Wuhan Diary*." *Cultural Politics*, Volume 17, Issue 1. Duke University Press, 2021. Pg. 74.

debate. In order for this to take place there were a series of pre-conditions that needed to be in place. The first such pre-condition was the massive readership that Fang Fang had built up over the course of her diary's 60-day run. As diary entries were transmitted through various online portals—these included blog-style posts on Weibo and WeChat—many entries were posted online through various websites and news portals as stand-alone articles, PDF compilations were shared through email and WeChat, and video streaming sites posted audiobook-style readings of entries. It is difficult to get an accurate tally of the diary's actual readership; however, we know that after just a few days of posting, early posts were generating two to three million hits online. That number quickly swelled to 10 to 20 million netizens reading each post within just days of being uploaded. Some estimates have claimed that, at the height of its popularity, many of Fang Fang's diary posts were garnering more than 50,000,000 readers in Chinese. To provide just one concrete example, one post from February 29, which was removed from the internet and later reposted through another account, received 800,000 views in just one hour. According to an article in *The Guardian*, as of April 10, "'Fang Fang Diary' has had 380m views, 94,000 discussions, and 8210 original posts"[10] and that was just on Weibo; the diary was also widely disseminated on WeChat and other websites and platforms. Multiple unauthorized audiobook versions appeared on YouTube, Bilibili, Youku, and other streaming sites. Passionate readers around the world began to translate passages into foreign languages and post them on social media; one Chinese-American high school student even started a website to post English translations of the diary.

Of course, during the height of the coronavirus outbreak there were many media outlets offering comprehensive coverage of the situation in Wuhan, from official state-run media like Xinhua News and CCTV to local newspapers, independent journalists, freelance photographers, video bloggers, and international media organizations. And unlike professional reporters who were "on the scene" offering reports from hospitals and profiles of frontline workers, Fang Fang was alone at home, quarantined in her apartment and observing the world through her window and the virtual windows of her cellphone and computer screen. **So what was it that allowed Fang Fang's voice to cut through all the noise and**

[10] Davidson, H. (2020). Chinese writer faces online backlash over Wuhan lockdown diary. The Guardian, April 10, 2020. https://www.theguardian.com/world/2020/apr/10/chinese-writer-fang-fang-faces-online-backlashwuhan-lockdown-diary

become, in the heart of so many readers, the voice of Wuhan? In the age of idol dramas, superficial consumption, and glossy celebrity culture, there were several factors that allowed Fang Fang to garner such a large and loyal readership. Firstly, there was a consistency to Fang's narrative. She posted each and every night, without fail, for 60 days. During a time riddled with uncertainties and questions, she was someone readers could count on. Her words could provide comfort and solace, and, over time, many readers projected an almost familial kinship relationship upon her. This attachment that so many millions of readers felt with the diary can perhaps be most powerfully demonstrated by the appearance of relay diaries, a phenomenon which Guobin Yang has discussed as follows:

> Fang Fang's diary was so popular that after she had written 60 entries and decided to stop writing in late March, her fans started a relay to carry on her cause. Reading Fang Fang's diary had become such a daily ritual in these diary communities that many found the absence of the ritual unbearable. So, they decided to write and post their own diaries as "relay diaries." From March 27 to May 29, 2020, 60 people wrote 60 "relay diaries" to match the number of Fang Fang's diary entries and continued their communal discussions in the comment sections of the diaries.[11]

These relay diaries are but one testament to the incredibly loyal reading community that Fang Fang's diary had nurtured over the course of its run. A second reason why so many readers gravitated to *Wuhan Diary* instead of the many other narratives available has to do with truth. Fang Fang's account was devoid of the propagandistic spin that reports by CCTV, Xinhua, and other state media outlets were inundated. She confronted the realities of life under lockdown with an unflinching frankness that did not shy away from discussion (and sometimes criticism) of COVID-19-related policies, but also took on issues of internet censorship, online trolling, discrimination, and the rise of political extremism. When the government performed well, she gave credit where credit was due, but she also did not hesitate when it came to calling officials out for mistakes and missteps. Unless you are a Chinese speaker who has lived within the

[11] Yang, Guobin. "In China, Pandemic Diaries Unite, and Divide, a Nation" in Social Science Research Council, Items, Insights from the Social Sciences, September 24, 2020. https://items.ssrc.org/covid-19-and-the-social-sciences/mediated-crisis/in-china-pandemic-diaries-unite-and-divide-a-nation/?fbclid=IwAR1HmfnaxGU2VLCxwhUc1lZ1p Ohn7RDXdH2WLXrhKfLL6XR7lZQ6TNs0piQ

Chinese-language media sphere for an extended period of time, it is hard to appreciate just how rare this is to encounter. But it was also precisely this unwavering commitment to truth that earned Fang Fang the trust, faith, and devotion of millions of readers. One of China's leading cultural critics and public intellectuals, Zhu Dake 朱大可 also singled out Fang Fang's commitment to documenting what really happened:

> She was there in the epicenter of the outbreak and, using a woman's sensitivity and her own unique breed of courage, used a completely public forum to try and document both her feelings and the reality of living amid a "besieged city"; she singlehandedly built a virtual "wailing wall" for all of us online and provided us with a luxury that is quite rare in China — truth.[12]

It was also in those rare passages where Fang Fang called for justice and accountability that her readers found a voice that was willing to fight for *them*. It should be noted that Fang Fang's criticisms of the government are always expressed from the perspective of a loyal and well-meaning citizen. If similar appeals had appeared in Europe or the United States, they would have likely garnered little attention, but context is everything. During the COVID-19 lockdown in Wuhan, Fang Fang's voice was enough to ignite a firestorm of debate, which is itself extremely revealing when it comes to gauging discourse and debate in contemporary Chinese society. Evidence of just how powerful this notion of Fang Fang's "truth" was can be seen in the later online attacks against her—one of the first things that was targeted was the diary's credibility.

At the same time, although Fang Fang may be a well-known writer who previously held the highest rank in the Hubei Writers Association, which is very much an "official appointment," *Wuhan Diary* is a document without pretensions. It is of the everyday, it is relatable. What Fang Fang describes is what millions of other Chinese citizens were also experiencing in real time; she was able to perfectly diffuse the fear, boredom, uncertainty, frustration, and anger of the lockdown in a way that allowed readers to see themselves through her words. And, finally, it is a document brimming with compassion and humanity. *Wuhan Diary* may be a portrait of a city during one of its darkest hours in its modern history, but, at its core,

---

[12] "Check Out Which Specialists Support Fang Fang and Who is Against Her" ("Kankan zhichi he fandui Fang Fang de zhuanjia dou you shei? 看看支持和反對方方的專家都有誰?) by Feng Yunkan https://zhuanlan.zhihu.com/p/133760882

it is also a love letter to Wuhan, an intimate testament to Fang Fang's relationship with this city. It is this combination of Fang Fang's reliability, sympathy, courage to speak truth to power, fight for the disenfranchised, and deep sense of humanity that allowed *Wuhan Diary* to transform into the literary and cultural phenomena that it became. At the same time, this massive following also precipitated its own downfall.

In China, any non-governmental organization with a large following, from churches to the once popular cult Falun Gong, can be perceived by the authorities as a potential threat. In the case of Fang Fang, the potential threat came closer to being realized through her repeated calls for "accountability." I would argue that her consistent cries for negligent officials to apologize and resign for missteps that had been taken were likely not seen as threatening so much for the specific cases she cited as for the *potentiality for amplification*. In other words, Fang Fang's single voice demanding that the Director of Central Hospital resign for negligence is one thing, but her 50 million readers rising up and making *other* demands was the x-factor, which could have potentially destabilizing repercussions. It was this potentiality for amplification which was an important factor contributing to the noisy response by ultra-nationalists.

Another crucial pre-condition that one needs to take into consideration in order to fully understand the evolution of the attacks against *Wuhan Diary* is the history of ultra-leftist groups attacking the author. The online attacks against Fang Fang did not suddenly materialize out of thin air during the coronavirus outbreak in order to target her diary. These attacks date back as early as 2017, beginning with *Soft Burial*, a novel Fang Fang first published in 2016. The novel explored the lingering trauma experienced by a family living in the long historical shadow cast by the Land Reform Movement. The Land Reform Movement was a political effort initially launched by Mao in 1946, and then, after the founding of new China in 1949, the campaign reached new heights, eventually lasting until 1953. It was regarded as an unmitigated success by the CCP, aimed at righting the exploitation and historical wrongs that generations of people had suffered under feudalism. According to official CCP historiography, the untold violence that was unleashed upon the landowning class was regarded as a historical necessity.

Unlike many earlier socialist literary works about the Land Reform Movement, which celebrated the victory of the exploited class over their oppressors, *Soft Burial* examined the trauma experienced by members of the land-owning class. Rather than a one-dimensional version of history,

2 VIRAL DIARY   23

Fang Fang's novel laid out the tensions, contradictions, and complexities of history and historical memory; it showed how singular acts of violence trigger inter-generational patterns of trauma and repression that last for decades. Ironically enough, one of the main plot devices of the novel revolves around a set of mysterious diaries locked away in an old trunk. The diaries belong to a victim of the Land Reform Movement and, decades after they were written, prove to be a crucial key for the victim's son to unlock the secrets of his family's traumatic past. *Soft Burial* was met with acclaim upon its initial publication. The novel was brought out by one of China's leading publishing houses, People's Literature, and in April of 2017 *Soft Burial* even won the prestigious Lu Yao Literary Prize. However, the day before the award ceremony for the Lu Yao Prize, a conference on *Soft Burial* was held in Wuhan. To call the meeting held that day a conference is something of a misnomer: it was actually more of a denunciation session that was highly reminiscent of the kind of campaigns against literary works held during the height of the Mao era. According to coverage of the event featured in *The New York Times*, at the meeting "Former Organization Minister of the Wuhan Steel Plant, Yin Xueyuan 殷學元, delivered a speech in which he accused Fang Fang of insulting and belittling the Land Reform movement with the intention of overthrowing the Chinese Communist Party. The conference even had a large banner hanging which declared '*Soft Burial* is a poisonous weed.'"[13] Additional attacks came in the form of a series of essays uploaded on May 22, 23, and 24 to the leftist (pro-CCP) website Red Culture Online (Hongse wenhua wang 紅色文化網) with titles like "*Soft Burial* is a Vindictive Counterattack Against the Land Reform Movement."[14] The essays alleged that Fang Fang, through the publication of a single work of fiction, was attempting to retroactively sabotage the historical legacy of the Land Reform Movement.

In the case of "*Soft Burial* is a Vindictive Counterattack Against the Land Reform Movement," the author, Zhao Keming 趙可銘, was actually

[13] Luo Siling 羅四鴒. "After Being Attacked by Leftists, Fang Fang Discussed the 'Soft Burial' of *Soft* Burial" ("Zaodao zuopai weigong zuojia Fang Fang tan ruanmai de ruanmai" 遭左派圍攻，作家方方談《軟埋》的"軟埋") in The New York Times Chinese Edition. June 27, 2017. https://cn.nytimes.com/china/20170627/cc27fang-fang/

[14] Zhao Keming 趙可銘. "*Soft Burial* is Vindictive Counterattack Against the Land Reform Movement" ("Ruanmai shi dui tugai de fangongdaosuan" 《軟埋》是對土改的反攻倒算) in Red Culture Online (Hongse wenhua wang 紅色文化網), May 25, 2017. http://www.hswh.org.cn/wzzx/llyd/zz/2017-05-22/44243.html

not a literary critic but a General in the Chinese army who formally served as Political Commissar at PLA National Defense University. The essay was written in a political style highly reminiscent of Cultural Revolution-era rhetoric and contained passages such as: "A negation of China's great Land Reform Revolution shall not be tolerated and the political mistakes of *Soft Burial* demand to be met with severe criticism."[15] Later in the essay, General Zhao even makes a series of concrete recommendations concerning the book, including "We must learn from the method of criticism employed by Comrade Deng Xiaoping 鄧小平 in the 1980s against *Unrequited Love* (*Ku lian* 苦戀), *River Elegy* (*He shang* 河殤) and other [ideologically] incorrect works…it is only through the process of going through criticism and compulsory thought struggle that we will achieve the goal of uniting the vast majority of writers and artists and educating the broad masses and the younger generation."[16] Just a few days later, on May 25, 2017, in response to the flurry of criticisms circulating about the book, *Soft Burial* was pulled from bookstores and listings for the book on online bookstore like Dangdang were deleted. The novel, which had been awarded a major literary prize less than a month earlier, was effectively banned.

The controversy, ultra-leftist attacks, and eventual suppression of *Soft Burial* are essential pieces of the puzzle when trying to understand the 2020 attacks that Fang Fang would suffer for *Wuhan Diary*. The way online trolling attacks function is such that once an individual becomes targeted, a network of websites and political groups are activated and a series of political talking points are drawn up. The target's social media feed is followed and as soon as questionable or controversial posts emerge, the trolling network is reactivated. In this case, *Soft Burial* not only resulted in Fang Fang being labeled a so-called enemy of the people but also effectively activated an infrastructure of ultra-leftist websites and individuals that were already closely following the author, ready to pounce on her for any future political or ideological infraction.

Of course, in order to understand the context of these types of attacks one has to further historicize the controversy, not just by looking at *Soft Burial* and Fang Fang's personal record as a target for ultra-leftist radicals, but also by examining the much longer history of cultural policies regarding literature in the PRC. It was in 1942 that Mao Zedong delivered his

---

[15] Ibid.
[16] Ibid.

"Talks at the Yan'an Conference on Literature and Art (在延安文藝座談會上的講話),"[17] where the ideological foundation behind all literary and artistic creation for the ensuing decades would be established. The talks were highly prescriptive, laying out a dogmatic formula for creative work that included the production of art produced for workers, peasants, and soldiers; art should convey clear black-and-white message easily discernable to all readers and audiences; the political function of art should take precedence above all else; and other forms of art deemed nihilistic, art-for-art's sake, escapist, and counter to the revolutionary line should be destroyed. The policies that spun out of the Yan'an talks would result in a creative culture where works of literature and art were deemed "correct" or "incorrect" in terms of their political content. During certain historical periods, like the Anti-Rightist Movement and the Cultural Revolution, the stakes could be quite high; works deemed "incorrect" were labeled as "poisonous weeds" (*du cao* 毒草), subjected to mass criticism, and authors/artists faced various forms of persecution. In some cases, artistic works even became the target for nationwide campaigns, such as Mao Zedong's 1954 attack on Yu Pingbo's 俞平伯 reading of *Dream of the Red Chamber* (*Hongloumeng* 紅樓夢), the persecution of Hu Feng 胡風 and the group of writers associated with him in 1955, or the sweeping 1966 campaign against Wu Han's 吳晗 play *Hai Rui Dismissed from Office* (*Hairui baguan* 海瑞罷官), which corresponded to the start of the Great Proletarian Cultural Revolution.

The era of dogmatic literary and artistic models seemed to retreat somewhat during the Reform Era under Deng Xiaoping; from the 1980s into the 1990s and 2000s, the work of artists and writers became increasingly market driven and the political imperatives from the age of high socialism began to fade. That said, over the course of the Reform Era, there were of course writers who would occasionally deviate from the script or cross lines into taboo political zones. Those who follow the contemporary Chinese cultural scene will remember the heated debate and eventual suppression of the 1988 television documentary series *River Elegy*, which was labeled "anti-communist" in the wake of the events of 1989; the fanfare surrounding Jia Pingwa's 賈平凹 1993 novel *The Ruined City* (*Fei du* 廢都), which was banned for 17 years due to sexually explicit

---

[17] McDougall, Bonnie S. *Mao Zedong's "Talks at the Yan'an Conference on Literature and Art: A Translation of the 1943 Text with Commentary."* University of Michigan, Center for Chinese Studies, 1980.

content; and even future Nobel laureate Mo Yan 莫言 who was subjected to severe political criticism over his 1996 novel *Big Breasts and Wide Hips* (*Fengru feitun* 豐乳肥臀). But none of those or any of the other works deemed "controversial" in Reform-era China were subjected to the kind of scrutiny, attacks, and widespread vilification that was reserved for Fang Fang. Part of this shift has to do with more stringent policies in policing cultural production since 2014. (Another crucial aspect of the shift would involve the successful harnessing of social media and online engagement, which will be discussed later.) With the political rise of Xi Jinping 習近平, many of the cultural policies from the Mao era were reinvoked. On October 14, 2014, Xi Jinping delivered his own set of "Talks at the Beijing Conference on Literature and Art (在北京文藝座談會上的講話)," a political gesture that aimed at cementing the ideological lineage between Mao and Xi and reminding China's creative community that the political mission of the arts was far from over. In fact, during the initial wave of criticism against *Soft Burial* in May of 2017, many of the articles criticizing Fang Fang did so within the framework of Xi's talks from 2014, which were used as ideological fodder against the book.

In his book *Why Fiction Matters in Contemporary China*, literary critic David Der-wei Wang has discussed Xi Jinping's call to writers, filmmakers, and other artists to "tell the good China story" (講好中國故事). Like Mao Zedong had done for an earlier generation, "Xi asked the newest generation of cultural workers to intertwine discipline and blessing, asceticism and aestheticism, self-denunciation and self-fulfillment, and this-worldly travail and the coming of utopia so as to describe and realize the Chinese dream."[18] The crux of the issue is tied to Xi's notion of historical truth and what this "good story" means. Turning back to David Wang:

> The issue of truth claims leads to the ambiguous connotation of the Chinese character *hao* 好 (good, correct, positive, or well) used to qualify Xi's story-telling. "Tell the good China story" can also be translated into either "tell the correct or right China story" or "tell the China story well." Therefore, depending on how *hao* is interpreted, Xi's slogan takes on a different charge: descriptive, interlocutory, imposing, or even imperative. The questions boil down to one: who gets the final say about the "goodness" of a story?[19]

[18] Wang, David Der-wei. *Why Fiction Matters in Contemporary China*. Waltham, MA: Brandeis University Press, 2020. Pg. 3.
[19] Ibid. Pg. 5.

A crucial prerequisite for understanding *Wuhan Diary*, the controversy surrounding the book, and the inner tension that plays out within its pages lies in the notion of the "good China story." *Wuhan Diary* is a text written by a former high-ranking government official—Fang Fang served for many years as the Chair of the Hubei Writers Association—with such credentials she would normally be considered an ideal candidate to tell the "good story, the right story, the *correct* story" about the novel coronavirus outbreak in Wuhan. The book, in part, does that. Fang Fang lauds the efforts of volunteers; she pleads with her readers to be patient, follow quarantine protocols, and cooperate with the government; and she repeatedly makes statements like: "I always stand on the same side as my government, cooperating with all official actions, helping the government in convincing people who are not quite on board with various policies, and aiding the government by consoling all those anxious citizens."[20] However, Fang Fang deviates from the script, in that her highly personal account is brimming with brutal honesty, cries for intervention, and discussions of various missteps, which include the early lag in making the outbreak public, the way whistleblowers were handled, early misinformation about the potential for person-to-person transmission, the way in which news early on was suppressed so as to not disturb high-level government meetings, and poor judgment in regard to the holding of large-scale public events just as the outbreak was raging. She also goes a step further and calls for the government officials responsible for these missteps to assume responsibility for their mistakes, apologize, and resign. It was these repeated calls for "accountability" which inevitably would prove most controversial and explosive. All of these latter aspects of the diary, of course, deviated from what many officials and readers deemed "the good story." When Fang Fang's detractors began to accuse her of spreading lies, heresy, and rumors, what we are actually witnessing is, in part, a breakdown between "the good story" and "the true story." After decades of emphasizing Mao's (and now Xi's) prescriptive formula for literature, "ideological correctness" has become conflated with "truth." Once *Wuhan Diary* was

---

[20] Fang Fang. *Wuhan Diary: Dispatches from a Quarantined City*. New York: HarperVia, 2020. Pg. 61. It should be noted that many of these passages that laud government policies appear in the diary immediately after passages in which she reports her online posts have been censored or removed. This puts those passages supporting the government in a more complex context, opening up multiple interpretive possibilities, that is, is this Fang Fang displaying a public show of "good behavior" after being "reprimanded" or, more plausibly, is there an implicit sarcasm in those passages?

deemed a political liability, the next step was an assault on its truth claims. What was unique in the case of Fang Fang's *Wuhan Diary* was that this deviation from the script would trigger a mass campaign waged on a scale unlike anything carried out against any single writer in decades.

Of course, "accountability" did not become a sensitive term overnight. Ever since the formative days of the CCP, there has been a thrust to "criticize" (*pipan* 批判) and silence writers and intellectuals who have dared to speak out and demand a greater level of accountability on behalf of the party: during the Yan'an period of the 1940s, the writer Wang Shiwei 王實味, author of "Wild Lilies" ("Ye bai hehua" 野百合花), "claimed moral and ideological autonomy within the communist movement to criticize abuses of power and to offer, publicly, alternative policies"[21] resulting in his purge and eventual execution in 1947; Lin Zhao 林昭 who spoke up during the 1957 Hundred Flowers Movement (百花齊放) through her "blood letters" only to be purged the following year during the Anti-Rightist Campaign; the reportage literature of Liu Binyan 劉賓雁 who exposed corruption and press control in the 1960s (earning him the label of "rightist") and, after rehabilitation, again exposed social injustices in the 1980s, earning himself the reputation of being the "conscience of China," only to be later labeled a "dissident" and spend his final years in exile in the United States; the scar literature movement (*shanghen wenxue* 傷痕文學) in the 1980s, which revealed the horrors of the Cultural Revolution but was shut down by Deng Xiaoping after cries for accountability were perceived as a threat to political stability; or even the case of Liu Xiaobo 劉曉波, a prominent intellectual and Nobel laureate who spent his final years in prison for co-drafting Charter 08, a document calling for political reform. While firmly entrenched in this tradition, Fang Fang's case also presented important deviations; she consistently cited PRC legal code to make her augments, using the very system she was critical of to frame her calls for accountability; but more important was the context: unlike earlier literary works that called for accountability, the nature of the internet in 2020 and unprecedented attention being drawn to the COVID-19 outbreak provided a seemingly limitless potential for the viral spread of *Wuhan Diary*.

Twenty-three years earlier, I had actually written my undergraduate thesis on the political campaign launched against Wu Han and his play

[21] Dai Qing 戴晴. *Wang Shiwei and Wild Lilies: Rectification and Purges in the Chinese Communist Party 1942–1944.* Routledge, 1993. Pg. ii.

Hai Rui Dismissed from Office. During those attacks, denunciation essays appeared in newspapers, "big character posters" were plastered everywhere, and even schoolchildren were mobilized to criticize and attack the author and his play, which was labeled a "poisonous weed." The attacks, which commenced in November of 1965, are often cited as a harbinger of the Cultural Revolution, which was officially launched in May of 1966. The Cultural Revolution would turn into a sweeping political movement that would paralyze China for a full decade, disrupting the economy, shutting down schools, and leading to the persecution of countless artists, writers, and intellectuals. Wu Han would die in prison in 1969, and his wife and daughter would also die as a result of the persecution they faced during the Cultural Revolution. There are, of course, fundamental differences between the campaign against *Hai Rui Dismissed from Office* and the situation surrounding *Wuhan Diary* 55 years earlier; however, there are also quite a few similarities: the protracted nature of each campaign; the use of Cultural Revolution-era terminology, iconography, and rhetoric against Fang Fang; the pervasive mobilization campaigns employed to slander, discredit, and attack the victims; and the "witch hunt" tactics utilized to target friends and family of the victim and silence voices of dissent. The attack on *Wuhan Diary* was, arguably, the single most focused and protracted campaign against a single literary work since the attacks on *Hai Rui Dismissed from Office* at the onset of the Cultural Revolution. But there were differences this time around: the backdrop of a global pandemic and trade war, the new digital tools available for disinformation and attacks, and the central place the issue of translation would play, hinting at the international stakes and the global dimension of the campaign that was to follow.

CHAPTER 3

Translation and the Virus

Aside from my "day job" as a professor and scholar of Chinese film and literature, I have worked as a freelance translator and interpreter for nearly a quarter of a century. Over that period, I have translated classic contemporary Chinese novels by writers like Yu Hua 余华 and Wang Anyi 王安憶 and a variety of other mediums, including screenplays, subtitles, short stories, interviews, and essays. I have had the honor of serving as an interpreter for some of the Chinese cultural world's greatest living figures, including Nobel Prize winning writers Mo Yan and Gao Xingjian 高行健; award-winning filmmakers like Xie Jin 謝晉, Zhang Yimou 張藝謀, Jia Zhangke 贾樟柯, and Hou Hsiao-hsien 侯孝賢; and actors like Zhang Ziyi 章子怡. Over the years I have often looked at the process of taking on the author's voice as a kind of performance and the act of translating/interpreting is almost like being an actor. In the words of veteran translator Suzanne Jill Levine, "…translation is: a creative mode of writing in which the translator takes on the voice of a foreign writer."[1] So much of what I do is suppressing my own ego and voice and becoming a vehicle for the artist's voice to shine through. It is about revealing the artists' literary sensibilities, nuanced language, and unique style. This is especially true when interpreting: you speak in the first person, assuming the rhythm and cadence of the speaker, and when the speaker says something in the

[1] Levine, Suzanne Jill. *The Subversive Scribe: Translating Latin American Fiction*. Dalkey Archive, 2009. Pg. 11.

© The Author(s), under exclusive license to Springer Nature Switzerland AG 2022
M. Berry, *Translation, Disinformation, and Wuhan Diary*,
https://doi.org/10.1007/978-3-031-16859-8_3

original language that makes the audience laugh or cringe, my interpretation aims to elicit the same response. For me, whether or not the audience laughs at the same beats in translation has always been the gold standard for a good interpreter. Yet no matter how faithfully we may mimic the words of the speaker, translation is always a performance. The words may spill from my mouth or pen, but they are never truly "my words." The ideological position a writer assumes is never my position, even if it might, at times, overlap with my own. As I embarked on the translation of *Wuhan Diary*, I had always taken this to be a basic, self-evident truth regarding translation. We are literary messengers. At the same time, as a full-time academic I have been fortunate in that the works I have translated have not been "works for hire" but rather literary works that I personally selected on the basis of their literary merit. In that sense, there is certainly a level of aesthetic and even ethical engagement in the selection process, especially in terms of those works of historical fiction and narratives of trauma, which have resonated with my own research. It was nevertheless unsettling when detractors of *Wuhan Diary* tried to project jingoistic assumptions onto my decision to translate Fang Fang's work (without having even read the actual translation or understanding the context that led me to this project). Some detractors of the book went so far as to invert the traditional relationship between translator and author; according to many of the attacks I received, I, the translator, was actually the "mastermind" or even "author" of the project and Fang Fang was a figurehead puppet. For decades, translators have fought for greater recognition and visibility, and now here was a strange case where the translator was not just "recognized" but his role was "overdetermined" in a twisted context that positioned me as culpable for the so-called ideological errors of the original work. Of course, one of my other literary sins was the very act of translation itself. But over the course of the translation and the subsequent cyber campaign that targeted not only the book but the very *act of translation*, my views on the role of the translator would also begin to undergo a profound transformation. Was I simply an invisible messenger?

When I began translating *Wuhan Diary* I had just emerged from what had been the single most challenging translation project of my career. Over the course of more than two decades as a literary translator, I had consciously or unconsciously sought out literary works that would challenge me. Translating *Wild Kids* (*Ye haizi* 野孩子) during my first year of graduate school led me down a twisted labyrinth to track down obscure quotes, political references, and slang terms; *The Song of Everlasting Sorrow* (*Chang hen ge* 長恨歌), which I co-translated with Susan Chan Egan, was an epic narrative spanning one woman's journey through four decades of modern Chinese history while experimenting with free indirect discourse, essayistic-like prose passages, and a narrative strategy that intentionally eschewed macro-historical events in order to focus on the everyday. But *Remains of Life* (*Yusheng* 餘生) pushed me even further. It was an avant-garde novel that explored the aftermath of a violent indigenous uprising in 1930 Taiwan, which resulted in a swift and brutal crackdown on the part of the Japanese colonial powers. Vacillating between ethnographic research, autobiographical self-reflections, and fantastical fantasies imbued with sex and violence, *Remains of Life* was composed in an almost stream-of-consciousness style with no paragraph breaks and unconventional use of punctuation; it employed smatterings of Japanese, Taiwanese, and the indigenous Seediq language and featured a highly non-conventional structure. I worked on and off on the novel for nearly 15 years before it was finally published in 2017.

I have to admit that emerging from that experience made the thought of translating *Wuhan Diary* feel like a breath of fresh air, at least in terms of language. The samples I had read were straightforward, written in conventional prose, and deeply connected with the world we were living in. If *Remains of Life* was a wild and fevered dreamscape from another land, *Wuhan Diary* was a clear photograph from the here and now. There was something attractive about tackling a project like *Wuhan Diary*; it really felt like, after swimming through a dark swamp with weights tied to my arms and legs, I was now able to glide through pristine waters, unfettered and free, or so I thought. I was also eager to translate more works by female writers. Previous to this, I had only translated one novel by a woman writer (*The Song of Everlasting Sorrow* by Wang Anyi), as opposed to four novels by male writers. In the wake of the #MeToo movement, I had also begun to reflect more on the implicit biases we replicate through the authors we teach in the classroom and, in the case of my translation activities, the writers whose work we make available to the world. When I decided to collaborate with Fang Fang on *Soft Burial*, those issues were weighing heavy on me and had a direct impact on my decision to take on that project. But consciously or unconsciously, I'm sure that another central factor that drew me to *Wuhan Diary* was Fang Fang's rendering, in real time, of personal and collective trauma.

Although the technical challenges presented by *Wuhan Diary* paled in comparison to *Remains of Life,* Fang Fang's diary presented an entirely new set of hurdles to face, many of which were quite unexpected. The first challenge was simply a test of endurance. Because of the timely nature of the content, the US publisher HarperVia wanted to get the diary into readers' hands as quickly as possible. They set a firm deadline of April 15 for me to deliver the final manuscript, a mission impossible for a single translator. The source text was, quite literally, still being written and we did not have a final word count for the book's length. Based on the author's initial estimation of how many days she would write for, which I multiplied by the average word count of early entries, I estimated a complete manuscript of approximately 90,000 words. Completing a manuscript of that length in just seven weeks was already a tall order and would require me to translate at least 2000 words a day in order to stay on schedule. However, practical circumstances made things even more difficult.

First off, the length of the diary entries continued to expand as Fang Fang got closer to the end of the diary with many of the final entries being more than double the length of the early entries. Fang Fang also extended the scope of the diary. Initially we thought the diary might cover around 40 days; she eventually announced it would stop at 54 days, but ended up extending it to 60 days. This meant that what was originally estimated to be a 90,000-word text expanded to over 133,000 words. After an incredibly productive initial two weeks, my translation schedule was further stressed when I fell ill in early March. I had many of the symptoms of COVID-19 and thought of the irony of translating a book about the coronavirus as I fought that very disease. Thankfully, my COVID-19 test was negative and I was eventually able to get back to work, but I had lost a full ten days of precious work time as I nursed a fever, exhaustion, diarrhea, and shortness of breath. Given the inaccuracy of many early COVID tests, I continued to wonder if I had, in fact, been infected. By the time I had sufficiently recovered, I needed to translate between 4000 and 5000 words a day in order to complete the translation and rough copyediting before the deadline. For that final month, between mid-March and mid-April, I juggled this translation schedule with 24/7 childcare (by that time, my two elementary school-age children were taking all of their classes at home online) and my own 250-student course on Chinese Pop Culture at UCLA, which had also transitioned online. I worked up to ten hours a day, seven days a week, frequently staying up until the early am hours and waking at 6:00 am to resume, so I could squeeze in a little more work before my kids woke up, all the while constantly texting back and forth between Fang Fang, our agent, and the publisher. It was the most singularly intense and focused experience of my translation career and it taught me a new appreciation for both the craft and the importance of engaging with topics that have social impact.

Naturally, the unique circumstances of the book's production also impacted the translation in important ways. Initially fueled by adrenaline and a passion to contribute something to an important dialogue playing out around the world, by the end of the process, I was pushing through, just trying to make it to the finish line. The incredibly challenging work schedule had begun to take a toll on my health; my normally 20/20 vision was getting fuzzy; the tendons and muscles in my hands and arms were in constant pain from the inordinate amount of typing and I needed to wear wrist braces. All the while, I made sure never to sacrifice quality or take shortcuts that might compromise the literary integrity of the work; however, I knew there were details that were inevitably impacted by the schedule. The final book contained more than two dozen endnotes that I hastily added as I translated; I would have liked to have added another dozen more; I proofread the entire manuscript several times, but in an ideal world I would have read it a few more times. Most importantly, sometimes, you need some distance from a translation before releasing it to the world: to mull over word choices, play with alternative phrases to find the perfect rendering, and tweak lines of poetry. But in this case, there was little time for any of that. In some sense, this perhaps complemented Fang Fang's original literary vision: the diary was not a well-manicured masterpiece that was carefully revised and tweaked, but instead had an explosive quality. *Wuhan Diary* is a book of the moment, exposing the author's thoughts, fears, reflections, and emotions raw and in real time. In some sense, perhaps it made sense that the translation would also have a bit of that same rough edge to it.

Then, during the final stretch of the translation in early April, I faced a new series of challenges. As the book came under attack it became clear that the translation would be held up under a linguistic and ideological microscope, scrutinized to a degree unlike anything else I had ever translated. As I discuss in the next section, when even the book's title is subjected to unprecedented examination, one could only imagine what the trolls would do to the actual content of the translation. As the online attacks grew, I knew that this translation would be held to a very different standard than other works in translation about China, but even I was unprepared when a friend leaked a memo to me that seemed to lay out a plan to attack weaknesses in my translation as a strategy for suppressing the book. The memo came from a private individual who previously served as China Consultant to the World Federation of Advertisers. The letter, which was addressed to "Esteemed Comrade Leaders," frames itself as a "recommendation during a state of emergency":

> Under the current dire circumstances as the world battles this virus, I offer the following emergency recommendation to the motherland: During this critical moment as the anti-China forces are actively searching for proof to force Chinese to pay reparations, the western publication of Fang Fang's diary will massively increase the sway of their negative coverage about China. It will become a powerful piece of evidence to serve the international movement that hopes to punish the Chinese people and hold them accountable for the virus.
>
> There are cultural differences between China and the West and, in the eyes of Western readers, Fang Fang's diary will become an extremely dangerous snake in the grass, capable of threatening our national security.
>
> This is a matter of critical importance and I humbly request that national organs (or perhaps we can reach out to the Ministry of State Security or the Department of Discipline Inspection) to seek out Fang Fang herself and request that she immediately halt publication and distribution of her book. Specialists within these organizations can also analyze the translation of Fang Fang's diary in order to find flaws in the translation which can be quickly utilized in order to halt publication and foreign rights sales.
>
> [...] We will be able to find many deficiencies in the "translation" and it only takes one to provide rationale for halting publication.
>
> [...] I have a decade of experience working in the publishing field; if the country needs my help I am willing to participate in this battle.[2]

I remember feeling a chill run down my spine as I read this letter, which also recalled how the letter writer had successfully used this tactic in suppressing publication of a previous book. As a professor who has taught college-level courses on translation for 20 years, I am quite familiar with "close readings" of translated works, analyzing different translations to critique their accuracy, readability, and aesthetic choices, but this was

---

[2] This letter was provided to me by a credible source; however, in order to protect the identity of the source and the original author, I am withholding those names here.

something very different. This was a call to mobilize specialists to meticu-lously dissect a translation with the nefarious intention of suppressing a book's publication. Of course, this was not a "government policy" but a private letter written by one individual with "recommendations"; there is no way to know how widely disseminated the letter was or what the ulti-mate response to this memo was, but just the knowledge that people were reacting to the impending publication with these types of insinuations was already a sobering indication of the coming storm. When I received a copy of the letter it was already close to mid-April and the translation was nearly complete. However, the memo made me keenly aware of the fact that not only was the book being attacked, but the translation itself was also to be targeted and highly subjective topics of "loyalty to the original" and "accuracy," which are normally reserved for academic articles and book reviews in translation studies, were actively being considered for weapon-ization. Suddenly I was also struck by a Kafka-esque sense of paranoia; there was something completely surreal about the fact that there might be individuals who would be scrutinizing my translation with the specific intention of finding faults and errors in order to launch a larger campaign to discredit the entire book. In other words, questions of "loyalty" in the context of literary translation were to be used to question political "loy-alty" to a specific ideologically driven interpretation of reality.

I tried not to let the above memo, along with other online posts that seemed to echo similar sentiments, impact the translation process. My call-ing as a translator has always been to the integrity of the original work: an attempt to maintain loyalty to the content, style, and voice of the author above all else. Thankfully, by the time I was alerted to this "translation conspiracy," the bulk of the translation was already complete, but knowl-edge of what was happening did inject the feeling that there was a devil looking over my shoulder and it did impact the final book in subtle ways. Most notably, throughout the copyediting process, I was more inclined to err a bit heavier on the side of the "literal" as opposed to choices that would make the translation a bit more "free." One concrete example: Fang Fang's introduction was entitled *bingdu shi renlei gongtong de diren* 病毒是人类共同的敌人, which I translated as "The Virus is the Common Enemy of Humankind." My editor and I had discussed shortening the title to "The Virus is the Common Enemy" which rhetorically worked better and sounded much better to my ears. The omission of the subject "humankind" didn't bother me too much, since it is clearly stated in the actual text. This is the kind of minor translation decision I would normally make on the fly and feel comfortable with. It is a decision where a slight omission greatly improves readability, flow, and the aesthetic rhythm of the work in translation. However, given the unrealistic standard to "loyalty" that we knew critics of the book would hold us too, the editor and I exchanged several emails to discuss this; I even bounced the change by Fang Fang, who approved the revision as long as the essay proper, where the full sentence appears in context, still included "humankind." But, ultimately, we erred on the side of caution and stuck with the original full translation: "The Virus is the Common Enemy of Humankind." Another example included a handful of citations where Fang Fang mentions reading an unspecified "article online." In my first draft of the translation, I actually searched online and found the articles that Fang Fang had been referencing and slightly tweaked the text so that instead of the unspecific "I read an article online" I changed the text to read "I read an article on Xinhua" etc.; however, again, due to the overwhelming scrutiny the book was receiving, I decided to go back to the author's original more ambiguous rendering.[3]

The final challenge to the actual translation came with the first wave of online attacks aimed at me. I was less than a week away from completing the translation when the controversy surrounding the book's international release (to be discussed in more detail later) broke online. Suddenly, after weeks of blurry vision, carpal-tunnel-like hand and arm pain, exhaustion, and daily drama associated with changing deadlines and publication details, I was now a direct target. At the time, I wasn't entirely sure what the real motivation behind the onslaught of attacks was: was it an attempt

---

[3] Fang Fang did not significantly alter or edit the text of her diary before publication, but there were a few minor deviations between the diary text in its original blog format and the translated book version. Firstly, entries titled were used selectively in the original posts. Some included titles, others did not. For the final version of the book, Fang Fang decided that for the sake of consistency and readers' convenience, she would add titles for all entries in the diary. In the original diary, the word "Wuhan pneumonia" (Wuhan feiyan 武漢肺炎) appears three times; these occurrences were early on in the diary before novel coronavirus (xinguan bingdu 新冠病毒) was widely used. Due to the politicization of the terms "Wuhan Virus" and "Wuhan pneumonia," those mentions of "Wuhan pneumonia" received political scrutiny, and, after discussions with various officials in China, the author requested we remove that term from the book. In consultation with my editors, we agreed to honor Fang Fang's request and replaced "Wuhan pneumonia" with "New Virus" (xin bingdu 新病毒). Those were the only changes to the book's text that Fang Fang requested.

to intimidate me with threats so I would abandon the project? That was never on the table for me. But the attacks did serve as a psychological distraction during those final days of what was already an incredibly challenging translation project. It was almost as if they were trying to pull me off my horse and into a muddy quagmire of curses, lies, and disinformation. I tried as best as I could to ignore the noise and push through. I completed the translation on April 15, 2020, just three weeks after Fang Fang had written her final entry; meanwhile, a storm of hatred and vile attacks was just beginning to brew on the Chinese internet.

CHAPTER 4

Attack the Title

Part of that coming storm involved the title of the book. As mentioned earlier, I never imagined I would one day devote a short chapter to how a book title was rendered in English. But as I became involved with this project, I quickly learned that there was nothing typical about *Wuhan Diary*, not even the book title. In fact, among the wave of online attacks waged in early mid-April 2020, the book title was one of the primary topics singled out by the online trolls. It is partially in response to those attacks that I here document the process of how the book's title was selected and how it later became the target of politicized attacks. Along the way, I hope this also provides unique insights into how translators navigate seemingly mundane questions like: "how to render a book title?" When Fang Fang first agreed to allow me to translate her work on February 24, the diary was not only incomplete but it didn't even have an official title. Fang Fang's writings on the novel coronavirus outbreak had frequently been referred to as *Fengcheng riji* 封城日記, "Diary from a Quarantined City" or "Lockdown Diary"; some were also referred to the blog as *Fang Fang riji* 方方日記, or "Fang Fang's Diary."

Just a few days after producing a few sample chapters to show prospective publishers, I started playing with different potential English-language book titles. On February 29, I wrote to my agent:

...do you mind if I bounce some book title ideas off you? The original Chinese title of Fang Fang's book translates literally as "Diary from a

Quarantined City" but that feels a bit clunky to me. I have been using "Wuhan Diary" but "Quarantine Diary" could also work. Other possibilities could be "Notes from a Quarantined City" "Quarantine Notebook", etc... anyway, before I fully embrace "Wuhan Diary" I wanted to see if you have any strong opinion either way.

She liked "Diary from a Quarantined City," partly because of the way it resonated with Daniel Defoe's *A Journal of the Plague Year*. After refining the title and further experimenting with other options, I came up with a short list that included:

> *Wuhan Diary*
> *Diary from a Quarantined City*
> *Wuhan Quarantine Diary*
> *Wuhan Diary: Reflections from a Quarantined City*
> *Diary from a Quarantined City: Wuhan During the Coronavirus Outbreak*

I circulated the list to Michael Emmerich, a trusted friend and colleague who is also a prolific translator of Japanese literature, and he preferred the final option, which was also my early favorite. In fact, the earliest version of the sample chapters I produced carried the title *Diary from a Quarantined City: Wuhan During the Coronavirus Outbreak*.

Coincidently, just as I was bouncing ideas for the English title off friends and colleagues, halfway across the globe, Fang Fang was also refining the Chinese title. On February 29—the same day I emailed my agent and Michael Emmerich about the title—she texted me and told me that she had decided to use *Wuhan fengcheng riji* 武漢封城日記, a word-for-word translation would read as "Wuhan Quarantine City Diary," as the official Chinese title for the book.

Over the course of the next few days, Fang Fang and I would exchange over two dozen texts about the title of the book. She was pushing for a fairly literal translation of *Wuhan fengcheng riji*, something like "Wuhan Quarantine Diary" or "Wuhan Lockdown Diary" which aesthetically felt a bit flat in English. After *Diary from a Quarantined City: Wuhan During the Coronavirus Outbreak* didn't seem to receive an enthusiastic response from the author, I started re-thinking the title. The new direction was for something more streamlined and snappy, like "Quarantine Diary" or "Wuhan Diary." After more texts back and forth, we eventually settled on *Wuhan Diary*. I explained to Fang Fang that sometimes titles that sound great in one language just don't have the same poetic force in another. I gave the example of a novel I had translated 15 years earlier, Ye Zhaoyan's 葉兆言 *Yijiusanqinian de aiqing* 一九三七年的愛情 (literally: "The Love of 1937"), which I translated as *Nanjing 1937: A Love Story*. The original title sounds great in Chinese, but falls flat in English, which is why I tweaked it a bit, eventually adopting a revised title that captures the sensibility of the original but also works well in English. By early March, versions of the manuscript that were circulated to publishers were all simply titled *Wuhan Diary*, no subtitle.

Once *Wuhan Diary* found a home with HarperVia, I moved full steam ahead on the translation work; early on there were no editorial discussions regarding the title or subtitle that I was involved with. Eventually the editors at HarperVia started discussing a two-pronged publication strategy: there was a tentative plan to publish the first 40 days of the diary as a book first and then a full version at a later date, once the diary was complete. This was something of a contingency plan. At the time, Wuhan was still under lockdown, no one knew how long the coronavirus outbreak in Wuhan would last or how long Fang Fang would write for. It was at that time, around the end of March, that a new working subtitle crept in: "forty days under quarantine." Of course, the number "forty" was a placeholder; it might be 45 or 50, we just didn't know. Eventually, both the two-pronged publication plan (and that subtitle) would be abandoned as the outbreak in Wuhan started to come under control. Fang Fang started talking about bringing the diary to a close and a decision was made to publish the diary in one version in its entirety.

The first time the word "dispatches" entered our conversation about the book's title came via my editor at HarperVia. Because of the tight publication deadline, I had been sending my editor the translation in installments; on March 21 I sent a new installment to him and he responded a few days later on the 24th by saying: "After what's been happening in Europe and what seems to be about to happen in the States, Fang Fang's diary feels extremely urgent. I was rereading the entry about needing more facemasks and this time it hit me with a renewed intensity. It's like she is writing to us from the future. If we were publishing it today, we could add 'Dispatches from the Future' as a subtitle." I was also keenly aware of this sense that Fang Fang's writings were from the past but somehow showing us where things were going with the outbreak and, in that sense, very much felt like dispatches from the future. This notion of the book serving as a set of "dispatches" must have stuck with the editor because when we received the first version of the cover design, it contained a new subtitle: "Dispatches from the Original Epicenter."

While "Dispatches from the Original Epicenter" would not have been my first choice for a subtitle (I would have preferred something that contained the concept of "quarantine" in order to better convey Fang Fang's original vision), I did not object to the new subtitle. I thought it sounded fine, worked within the content and vision of the original book, and most importantly, I trusted the judgment of the editors at HarperVia when it came to how best to frame the book for mainstream English-language readers. I immediately shared the cover design with Fang Fang, which contained the new subtitle, but I did not discuss it with her at that point. This was an oversight on my part. At the time, besides corresponding with the author, various editors (there were around a dozen foreign language editions that had just been sold at that point), and agents dozens of times every day, I was also working at breakneck speed translating the book. Never in my wildest dreams could I have imagined that those five words— Dispatches from the Original Epicenter—would go on to unleash a maelstrom of politicized attacks and online fury.

Just a few days after seeing the cover design and new subtitle, the publisher's sales department uploaded a description of the book, the cover design (including the new subtitle), and other details to Amazon, Barnes & Noble, and other online book vendors. At that time, neither Fang Fang nor I had seen the description that was uploaded and Fang Fang had not realized that there was a new subtitle that the editors had added to the title. I never read this oversight as anything nefarious; the simple fact was that this entire book project was on a rush schedule, and everyone was doing their best to get the book out as soon as possible due to the importance of the subject matter. The coronavirus was coming and this was one of the first and most important early documents about the outbreak in Wuhan. What started as a project to raise awareness of what was happening in China became a desperate attempt to warn those of us outside China of what was coming to our shores. In that process, certain aspects of the production process were streamlined and details like vetting the book's description with the author were skipped.

Under normal circumstances, small details like the book's description would not be of great consequence, and, even if there were problems, we would still have plenty of time to revise before the official publication; the early text was more like a placeholder uploaded for online pre-sales in order to provide basic details about the book. But the circumstances in this case were far from normal. Somehow there was an unprecedented amount of scrutiny being placed on the international release of *Wuhan Diary*. I did not even know that the book's title and description had been uploaded online until I started to receive messages from Chinese readers who had read a version already translated into Chinese and posted on Weibo!

Having published more than a dozen books over the past 20 years, it is highly unusual to have a book's English-language description and title generate any attention in China, let alone be translated and widely discussed immediately after being uploaded. I realized that something was wrong—this book was increasingly becoming unlike any other typical publication. The first message about the subtitle that I received was from Professor M, a specialist in Translation Theory and Practice from S University in China. He emailed me on April 5 to state his objections to the subtitle, stating:

> the sight of the word 'original' in 'Dispatches from the Original Epicenter' printed on the cover of the advance edition has made me quite uncomfortable since that word is inevitably associated with the word 'origin'. As regards the origin of the virus, which is supposed to be a scientific issue, there is still much controversy and even political tension there. It had better be left to scientists. As you must be aware, meaning is constructed by the readership as much as, if not more than, it is meant by the author. Just imagine what the potential Chinese readers' emotional response to that ambiguous and therefore misleading 'original' will be like.[1]

Professor M.'s email came as a surprise; never before had I received an unsolicited email discussing the title of a book I translated, let alone the subtitle of a book months before it was even slated for release. At first I wasn't even sure if the email was an attempt to troll me, from a genuinely concerned reader, or a politically motivated attempt to interfere in the book's production. But one thing that had been taking place was, as I was busy spending up to ten hours a day translating *Wuhan Diary*, new debates had begun to emerge concerning "the origin of the virus." I had read a handful articles on this subject—some claimed that the novel coronavirus came from bats, others suspected it came from pangolins, some pointed to the Huanan Seafood Market, others to a virus created in a lab—but I did

---

[1] April 5, 2020, email from M. Name is here redacted to protect the privacy of the individual.

not have a position on this topic; it was naturally not something that fell within my field of expertise, nor was it a topic that Fang Fang discussed in her book. When I read the editor's subtitle, "Dispatches from the Original Epicenter," my reading was simply that this was a document attesting to and sending out messages to the world about what happened at the site of the first major outbreak of the novel coronavirus. Origins aside, Wuhan was indeed where we first witnessed large numbers of COVID-19 infections; that was the sole connotation of the title when I read it. At no point did I interpret the subtitle as an attempt to interject *Wuhan Diary* into the burgeoning scientific debates about the "origin" of the novel coronavirus.

However, I also realized that we were beginning to tread on complicated political terrain. In fact, discourse around the virus was transforming so quickly and dynamically that it started to feel like the tectonic plates were shifting beneath our feet. These shifts were not just taking place in China, but also in the United States, and many other countries around the world. The initial COVID-19 outbreak unleashed a wave of political radicalization that reverberated deeply, having a particularly explosive impact on Sino-US relations, which were already strained due to the ongoing trade war. Out of an overabundance of caution, I discussed the potential controversy that this new subtitle might elicit with my agent, the author, and the editors. When Fang Fang realized that a subtitle she never approved was being used, she immediately requested that it be changed. After some back and forth with the publisher, on April 8, they agreed to change the subtitle to "Dispatches from a Quarantined City," finally giving the book its final title: *Wuhan Diary: Dispatches from a Quarantined City*. It only took four days for the change to take place; however, it would take a bit longer for the new data (which also included a new description of the book, which had been approved by both Fang Fang and myself) to get uploaded to Amazon and other online sites. In the meantime, screenshots of the early title and book descriptions were spreading like wildfire on the Chinese internet and the fury was growing. What had initially felt like a minor bump in the road would turn out to be a boulder of Sisyphus.

The reason I have so painstakingly reconstructed the process by which we finally settled on a book title for *Wuhan Diary* is in order to adequately set the stage for what would come next. After more than a month of back and forth exchanges regarding the book's title, just as we had finally settled on *Wuhan Diary: Dispatches from a Quarantined City* as the official title, the book's previous working title of *Wuhan Diary: Dispatches from the Original Epicenter* (which was not unproblematically translated into

Chinese as 來自疫情源頭的報道) was still circulating online and virtually each and every word from that title would come under scrutiny and be the subject of multiple rounds of online attacks. I have never seen a book title scrutinized to the degree that *Wuhan Diary* was placed under an ideological microscope during the months of April and May of 2020.

The first round of attacks launched against the book's title began with the term "original epicenter," which was part of the book's early subtitle. This was one of the more vehement components of the early criticisms that were waged online. The email I had received back on April 5 expressing concern over the relationship between the terms "original" and "origin" prophetically indicated the first strike. In order to best sum up the nature of these attacks, I will quote from some of the Weibo users who came out publicly against the use of "original epicenter" and alleged that it was an attempt on the part of the author and translator to politicize the book. One Weibo user posted on April 20, 2020:

> The subtitle for the English edition of Fang Fang's Diary ---Dispatches from the original epicenter. The word "original" in this subtitle when used as an adjective it means "the first, the beginning, the earliest," but when used as a noun, it means "origin or where something comes from." Using such a term in the subtitle is extremely misleading, it is easy for people to come away with the impression that Wuhan is the site where the novel coronavirus originated from. However, even today scientists are still harboring doubts about [where the virus actually originated from]. By Fang Fang rushing to conclusions on the cover of *Wuhan Diary* she is in fact helping the Western Anti-China powers by offering China up to be attacked!

These comments are quite representative of what hundreds of other critics were also posting around this time. In fact, many of these posts use almost identical language and descriptions. A lot of the controversy arises from an issue of translation and interpretation. It is likely that the majority of the posts attacking the title were not written by English speakers and many were relying upon the literal Chinese translations floating around the internet, which definitively interpreted the subtitle as taking a political stance on the origin of the virus. The fact that many of the attackers were nonnative English speakers relying upon Chinese-language commentaries which politicized the subtitle also made it easy to manipulate the facts and push the "origin" reading of the subtitle. While I did not write the controversial subtitle, at no point was that my interpretation of the phrase.

Instead, I read the subtitle as indicating that Fang Fang's blog entries were coming from the site of the first major outbreak of the novel coronavirus: a fact that I don't think anyone could dispute.

There were of course some Weibo users who tried to offer a more nuanced and fair-minded reading of the controversy. One such interpretation came from Weibo user Qu Weiguo 曲衛國 who on April 9, at the very height of the attacks, posted the following:

> One of the reasons these people are so angry has to do with the subtitle of the English translation containing the words "the original epicenter," which they have definitively interpreted as meaning that China is the source of the virus. You need to have some foundation in English to recognize the word "original," but this term has multiple meanings including both the site of origin and the place where something first happened; "epicenter" simply means the center. Not long ago Italy followed China in becoming the epicenter of the pandemic, and now the United States is becoming the new epicenter. Wuhan was the site of the earliest large-scale outbreak of the coronavirus, the entire city was shaken to its core, so what is problem with this statement? Even CCTV stated similar things: "China paid a massive price in terms of the sacrifices we made in order to serve as the first line of defense against this virus for the world." What do you think they meant when they said "first line of defense?" If it hadn't first occurred here, how could we have been the first line of defense? These people seem to be patriots, but actually they are trying to kill the incredible contributions that the people of Wuhan and the people of China have made during their early battle against the virus. If we follow the logic of those critics, even CCTV news is fake and the first line of defense against the virus was never even in China.
>
> One of the reasons for their anger is that they think that Fang Fang's Diary is going to be used by the anti-China faction in the West as a tool to smear China and later serve as evidence for them to exact reparations from China. It is impossible that they are completely ignorant when they make these statements. But this typically shows just how they are utterly devoid of faith they are in this great nation of China. Do they really think that 60 installments from a diary that has been circulated online will bring China to its knees? Will it be able to provide evidence that China is the source of this virus? It is, in fact, their state of utter fear that will show those anti-China elements just how weak China really is.

Unfortunately, while more level-headed views, like those of Qu Weiguo, can be found online, his comments were in direct response to the deluge of views posted around April 9, which presented the reading of the initial subtitle in an overwhelmingly negative and politicized framework. More typical responses to the subtitle include this post from April 8:

> Is Fang Fang's quarantine diary a dispatch from the original epicenter? Congratulations to the Western media for getting your hands on some new material that will allow you to demonize China at an even more fevered pitch! Is the Western media going to assert that *Wuhan Diary* provides irrefutable evidence to exact reparations from the Chinese people? If this diary, which is filled with rumors and hearsay, fans the flames of anti-Chinese sentiment, what kind of terrible situation will the millions of overseas Chinese be left in? This will only help the United States in its scheme to use the virus to vilify China.

Another example can been seen in this post from April 10 by another Weibo user: "Look at this book title; the devious cunning of this wolf is now revealed for all to see—the American imperialists' evil plot to sully the good name of China and Wuhan has now been revealed in Fang Fang's grotesque and contemptable act of national betrayal!" The post also included an unflattering photo of Fang Fang next to a separate image of Donald Trump with the meme "You people just wait and see!". During the period April 8 through mid-April, posts, articles, and messages like this one from ZDW would inundate Weibo. Even after the book's subtitle was officially changed to *Dispatches from a Quarantined City*, attacks on the now-obsolete subtitle continued. One post from May 15, the publication date of e-book version in the United States and the United Kingdom, erroneously claimed: "It has been many days now since Fang Fang's *Wuhan Diary* has been published abroad and now foreigners can easily purchase this book which publicly claims that the novel coronavirus originated in China...." Even in May 2021, more than 13 months after the subtitle had been changed, attacks on the "original epicenter" tagline were still appearing on Weibo.

As unprepared as I was for the series of attacks on the phrase "original epicenter," I was even less prepared for the series of posts that would follow. Given the way in which the controversy and various global conspiracy theories around the epidemiological origins of COVID-19 had been gaining traction, I could understand how the words "original epicenter" could be twisted to be construed as meaning something very different than what was originally intended—that is precisely why we pushed to have the phrase removed—however, what came next was even more tendentious.

Some Chinese readers began to latch onto the word "dispatches" and, sharing screenshots from Chinese-English dictionary pages featuring the definition of the term, homed in on the fact that the term is frequently used to describe telegrams or urgent messages sent by international journalists, military officers, or other government officials stationed abroad. From these definitions came allegations that Fang Fang was working against China as an agent for a foreign government. By the end of April, Fang Fang's name was frequently appearing on Weibo with the new title "Special Correspondent Fang Fang" (Fang Fang tepaiyuan 方方特派員), which was used by her detractors in a way that held close connotations to the label "special agent" in Chinese. What all of these politicized and overly literal interpretations missed was the simple fact that the subtitle—whether it be the original "Dispatches from the Original Epicenter" or the later final version "Dispatches from a Quarantine City"—points to something else entirely. These are dispatches from a place where, at least when Fang Fang began writing, very few people in the world understood what was happening there, and more importantly, they were dispatches from a place that foretold our common fate as COVID-19 spread globally. In contrast to the conspiratorial readings of "dispatch," I much prefer Kevin Robin's reading of the term in the context of *Wuhan Diary*:

> They were dispatches, precisely – and dispatches on anything and everything, from online shopping tips to care for the lives and well-being of those afflicted by the coronavirus illness. The whole phenomenon – actually, we should be thinking of it as an online media event – was a vast exercise in writing, cutting, pasting, forwarding, and circulating of texts, messages, photos, and video clips, and increasingly included feedback and participation from millions, literally, or readers and followers.[2]

"Dispatches" may not have existed in the original Chinese title, but in the context of a book now being marketed to international readers, the connotations made perfect sense. It should also be noted that adding a subtitle to the English edition of an international title is not at all unusual: in fact it is extremely common. (Subtitles were added to the titles of all five of the Chinese novels I previously translated, even though none of them had a subtitle in the original.)

---

[2] Kevin Robins. "The Great City is Fragile: Fang Fang's *Wuhan Diary*." *Cultural Politics*, Volume 17, Issue 1. Duke University Press, 2021. Pg. 70.

After attacks on the words "original epicenter" and "dispatches," next came Wuhan. When the diary first began gaining attention in China, it was most commonly referred to as "Quarantine Diary" (*Fengcheng riji* 封城日 記) or simply "Fang Fang's Diary" (*Fang Fang riji* 方方日記). It was only when pre-sale information for the English and German editions of the book appeared online in early April that "Wuhan Diary" emerged as the official title. When the word "Wuhan" began to come under attack by Chinese online trolls, a true sense of the surreal took over. What could possibly be problematic with the name "Wuhan"? Yet in late April a new torrent of posts began to appear on Weibo with statements like: "I just want to ask that animal that wrote that diary, what right does it have to call the book *Wuhan Diary*?" (4/29/20), while another user wrote "I never read *Fang Fang's Diary* but I felt extremely uncomfortable when I heard that they changed the title to *Wuhan Diary* for the foreign edition." Another post rhetorically asked: "Who is this Fang Fang person? What right does she have to write a *Wuhan Diary*? I have no idea who Fang Fang is, but because of all the controversy and heated debates this year, I learned that this Miss Fang Fang wrote a book called *Wuhan Diary*. My first impression is: Does Wuhan really need a diary?" (7/13/20). The main thrust of these and countless other posts is that Fang Fang does not have the right to speak for or represent the citizens of Wuhan, let alone the city itself. Of course at no point in the book does Fang Fang claim to do that; in fact, she repeatedly encourages her readers to write and publish their own diaries and narratives about what they are experiencing during the coronavirus outbreak. As Fang Fang observes, "one person's document is never enough; it can never capture the entire picture, but when you collect countless individual records together, you can begin to get a more complete picture that represents the truth of what happened."[3]

Finally, even the word "diary" was under attack. In another attempt to attack the book, even the author's chosen literary form was scrutinized in order to further undermine the very legitimacy of *Wuhan Diary*. Although the Chinese term *riji* 日记 while most commonly translated as diary can also be rendered as journal or even record or notebook, Fang Fang's writings began to be referred to as a "diary" in English-language media even long before the English translation was announced. At one point in early May, shortly before the e-book publication, a longtime friend who works

---

[3] Fang Fang. *Wuhan Diary: Dispatches from a Quarantined City.* New York: HarperVia, 2020. Pg. 212.

as a career translator at the United Nations sent me a gentle message suggesting I replace "diary" with the term "journal"—he had been following the controversy online and already anticipated that the term "diary" might elicit additional attacks. We stuck with diary party because it would have been too late to change the title again (we had just revised the subtitle) and the work was already widely referred to in both Chinese and Western media accounts as a "diary"; at the same time, it started to feel like the paranoia surrounding the book had grown out of control; we needed to draw a line. So the title *Wuhan Diary* stood unchanged, but eventually, as my friend predicted, even the term "diary" came under scrutiny. A small fraction of the posts criticizing Fang Fang's positioning of the book as a diary included comments like:

> Fang Fang's Diary includes so many 'my friend said,' my doctor friend said,' 'a friend online said,' and phrases like 'possibly; and 'perhaps' and other forms of hearsay as she sat at home in Wuhan took in all these things she purportedly heard --- can you call that a diary? Shouldn't a diary be about one's own experiences? (4/10/20)

> You shouldn't call a record of things you never experienced a diary, instead this pile of messed up garbage and fabricated rumors should be called 'Fang Fang's Sexual Fantasies'! (4/22/20)

> Chairman Wang's [alluding to Fang Fang's real name, Wang Fang] Wuhan Diary shouldn't be called a 'Diary.' It would be much better if they called it 'Rumors I Heard and Embellished.' (7/23/20)

The greatest irony is that the term diary was not even a term consciously employed by Fang Fang, but given by her readers. As Fang Fang explained, "Some of the more enthusiastic readers even collected all of my posts into digital files and renamed them 'Fang Fang's Quarantine Diary.' That is how people started referring to the collection as a 'diary.'"[4]

Earlier I discussed Lu Xun's "A Madman's Diary," a revolutionary text that helped launch the modern Chinese vernacular literature movement, and, over the decades, there have been many other important Chinese literary texts written in the diary format—like Ding Ling's 丁玲 1928 canonical work of fiction "Diary of Miss Sophia" ("Shafei nushi riji" 沙菲

[4] Fang Fang. "I Will Face it All with No Misgivings: After *Wuhan Diary*" in *Wuhan Diary: Dispatches from a Quarantined City*. Revised Paperback edition. HarperVia, 2022. pg. 362.

女士的日記)—but perhaps the most widely read diary of the twentieth century in China was *The Diary of Lei Feng* (*Lei Feng riji* 雷鋒日記). Written by a model soldier who spent his days studying the work of Mao Zedong and doing good deeds, the diary was published posthumously in 1963. *The Diary of Lei Feng* contains extensive passages documenting the author's selflessness, frugality, and attempts to internalize the lesson that one should be content to be a cog in the machine. *The Diary of Lei Feng* was a very different form of "diary"; it was a political text, a handbook of proper behavior, and public testimony of political allegiance to Chairman Mao and the party. Perhaps this was the criteria the Fang Fang's detractors were using to appraise her diary? Looking at *Wuhan Diary* from this perspective, Fang Fang's account certainly did not conform to the political prescription of what a "proper diary" should be.

Of course, from Lu Xun to Ding Ling and from Lei Feng to Fang Fang, each of these diaries was written against a very different historical backdrop, engaged with different literary forms (including allegory, fiction, propaganda, and exposé), was disseminated in different ways (literary journals, book form, state-sponsored propaganda networks, and the internet), and had radically different intended readerships. That said, the controversy surrounding the nomenclature of "diary" is certainly tied in part to this earlier literary history of the diary as a genre in modern China, with claims that Fang Fang's account was "fiction" pointing back to the tradition of Lu Xun and Ding Ling and other criticisms that the diary failed to adequately champion the party line, harkening back to the kind of "model diary" embodied by *The Diary of Lei Feng*.

But perhaps for the biggest literary clue on the ethical role that the diary form should play in society, we should turn to none other than Fang Fang herself. In her controversial 2016 novel *Soft Burial*, the protagonist Qinglin grows up with little knowledge of his parents' mysterious family background: he never had any relatives growing up, his father died when he was still a child, and his mother suffered from a strange form of memory loss. The only clue to Qinglin's past is found locked away in an old trunk containing his late father's diaries and it is there in those old tattered pages, unread for decades, that the protagonist learns of the trauma and pain his parents experienced. (Both of Qinglin's parents were victims of the Land Reform Movement and assumed new names and identities to survive after their families were killed.) After a long journey to dig deeper into his family's history, Qinglin ultimately gives up; he locks the diaries back and up and decides it is better to let the past rest. But in the end, his professor friend, ultimately the moral conscience of the book, decides that the truth must be told. The diaries, which for Qinglin stand as a devastating wound, an unspeakable taboo that must be kept hidden, also represent a higher form of historical truth and are ultimately revealed. And it is in that final denouement that Fang Fang's ethical responsibility to witnessing and recording history, bearing testimony, and protecting truth, as painful and inconvenient as it might be, is fully revealed... and it all begins with a diary.

By the time the trolls began to target even the "diary" form of *Wuhan Diary*, it was clear that these attacks were not guided by logic or legitimacy, but instead an incessant ideological drive to tear the book down, no matter what the cost and no matter how tenuous the claims against it might be. At this point it was obvious that anything contained within the title would have received attacks. The role of a book's editor is also worth pointing out as a crucial player whose contributions to a publication are often not understood or recognized. While thousands of online trolls attacked Fang Fang and me for the book's subtitle, we had in fact no role in drafting that first version which incited such ire; moreover, as soon as the author became aware of the content, she immediately demanded it be changed; yet in the eyes of millions of Chinese netizens, she would continue to bear the brunt of the responsibility. As for why an army of trolls would home in on the title and subtitle of the book, the answer is actually quite simple: that's all they had. The translation at this point had not even been published and there was no real content for the book's detractors to sink their teeth into and so an entire hate campaign was orchestrated around just the title of the book.

The strategy employed in the attacks against the book's early working title *Wuhan Diary: Dispatches from the Original Epicenter* and later official title *Wuhan Diary: Dispatches from a Quarantined City* was similar to the tactics first pioneered by former US junior senator Joe McCarthy in the 1950s during his attempt to turn the public against alleged communists. In the words of McCarthy's biographer, Larry Tye, speaking to NPR's Terry Gross:

> [McCarthy] played the press brilliantly. If you release your most damning information out in the hinterlands...the reporters were not going to know who to call at the State Department. They were not going to get the kind of responses you could hope for... Any responses would come tomorrow on page 24. He understood that if you lobbed one bombshell and that had

been proven to be a fraud, rather than waiting for the press the next day to expose it as a fraud, he had a fresh bombshell ready to go.[5]

Fast forward 70 years, the "hinterlands" has now been replaced with the virtual wild west of Weibo, a place where reputable news sources, rumors, lies, and disinformation are all seemingly democratized by the nature of the platform itself, appearing side by side in the news feeds of users and leaving readers on their own to separate the truth from the lies. But the platform is actually not democratic in that, thanks to aggressive censorship practices coupled with online bullying and intimidation, certain political perspectives receive privileged treatment over others. Attacks waged against Fang Fang's book were not being generated by official media sites like Xinhua or CCTV, they were from the accounts of thousands of individual Weibo users, making the source—much like the virus itself—difficult to track, trace, and fully understand. But even more telling is the strategy of lobbing one bombshell after another, a shock-and-awe technique, that leaves the target helpless to respond. It is like a cyber-media hydra; by the time you cut off one head, six more have already sprouted. And by the time that all of the words in the title and subtitle—Wuhan, diary, dispatches, original, epicenter—had been thoroughly attacked and exhausted, the book's detractors would move on to other aspects of *Wuhan Diary* that would be subjected to the ideological microscope and, in the process, weave a complex web of conspiracy theories to surround Fang Fang and her book.

[5] Terry Gross interview with Larry Tye on *Fresh Air*, July 7, 2020. https://www.npr.org/2020/07/07/887649136/we-ve-got-to-learn-from-our-history-demagogue-author-warns

CHAPTER 5

Unleash the Trolls

The cyber campaign launched against Fang Fang in 2020 was truly on an unprecedented scale. *Wuhan Diary* engaged tens of millions of readers and elicited intense and protracted engagement on various websites and social media platforms. **But what were these attacks actually focused upon? What did they look like? And how were they carried out?** The previously discussed overview of the controversy surrounding the title of the book provides a snapshot of but one aspect of how the book was targeted, but the full scope of the attacks extended much deeper and was much more complex. As Lai Fu 來福 has observed, in the beginning the "attacks on Fang Fang were quite predictable, falling back on talking points related to 'spreading rumors,' 'negativity,' and 'passing the knife'"[1]; however, over time they would expand to include broader accusations that included an attempt to inspire a "colour revolution" in China, that she was representing "foreign powers," and part of an "imperialist" plot.[2] Most of these online attacks against Fang Fang fell into one of five categories: (1) criticism that *Wuhan Diary* is based on hearsay/secondhand accounts, (2) attacks on the authenticity of the diary and the details of its

---

[1] Lai Fu 來福. "The Battle Over Fang Fang: Old Answers and New Questions to the 'Theory of Passing the Knife'" (Fang Fang Zhanzheng: Tidaolun dejiuda'an he xin wenti方方戰爭:「遞刀論」的舊答案和新問題) Initium Media, May 20, 2020. https://theinitium.com/article/20200515-opinion-fangfang-people-war-national-socialism/
[2] Ibid.

production, (3) criticisms of Fang Fang for allowing her diary to be published outside of China, (4) allegations that the diary was tied to one of several conspiracy theories, and (5) personal attacks. Of course, there were other attacks and accusations, but most of the online chatter concerning *Wuhan Diary* can fit into these categories, often with a certain degree of overlap.

Beginning with accusations of hearsay/secondhand accounts, these attacks took issue with Fang Fang's citation of sources. Throughout the diary, Fang Fang repeatedly refers to her friends, colleagues, neighbors, classmates, and, most often, "doctor friends." She relays phone conversations with them, quotes text messages they send her, and discusses topics that come up in chat groups with them. However, the vast majority of the time, Fang Fang does *not* identify these individuals by name. Withholding the identity of her "informants" earns Fang Fang the ire and scorn of her attackers. They claimed she was "spreading rumors," "basing her entire diary on hearsay," and equated her standards of accuracy to an "elementary school student diary."[3] Later parodies of the diary would also embellish this feature.[4] Fang Fang's decision not to reveal her sources reveals a few important truths about different literary forms; it is also illustrative of how individuals navigate a hostile world of online bullying and smear campaigns. Firstly, Fang Fang is writing a diary, presented albeit in an open online format, but a diary nevertheless. She is not a journalist, a correspondent, or the representative of an official news agency; she was writing from the perspective of an individual and there is therefore no rationale for holding her to journalistic standards when it comes to citing and authenticating sources. *Wuhan Diary*, in its original form, was essentially a blog, written daily in a raw and unedited form and immediately uploaded to the internet. That said, Fang Fang is a veteran writer who has published nearly a hundred books, including numerous non-fiction works on Wuhan cultural history; she is certainly well aware of proper citation practices. The real issue here is that this is a writer who, since 2017, has been consistently targeted by a virtual army of online trolls. Fang Fang was keenly aware

---

[3] Article originally posted to Weibo by Mr. Lu Guoping 魯國平先生. "Are we being too hard on Fang Fang by criticizing her diary as a work of 'hearsay'?" ("Zhize fangfang riji daotingtushuo shi keqiu ma" 指責方方日記 "道聽途說" 是苛求嗎?) April, 23, 2020. https://k.sina.cn/article_1142648704_441b6f8001900m7a6.html

[4] See the discussion of "American Diary" in the chapter The Strange.

that by revealing her sources she was most certainly putting them in a position of great vulnerability, opening them up to the very attacks she was receiving. Besides discussing this issue in numerous interviews on the public record, Fang Fang even directly addressed the question of withholding names in her diary proper:

> Speaking of "my doctor friend," I should make it clear that I have more than one. I should also tell Xiang Ligang 項立剛 and his cronies that these doctors are professionals at the very top of their fields; so I am certainly not going to publicly reveal their names. The reason I insist on withholding their names is precisely because dregs like you exist. Our mindless government might buy your one-sided stories, but I will never let my friends become your victims. This afternoon another doctor friend (a leading expert in his field, but, again, I cannot reveal his name) called me.[5]

More than anything else, the absence of proper names and full source citations should not be read as a "flaw" of the diary but a key characteristic, which through this absence bears witness to the precarious act of bearing witness. In other words, the inability of the writer to cite sources, name names, and give credit where credit is due speaks to the systemic flaws of a system where individuals live in fear of reprisals and online attacks by self-fashioned online nationalist vigilantes and the "human-flesh search" (*renrou sousuo* 人肉搜索) machine. Not only that, but the very act of protecting her sources then gets twisted by trolls into fodder to further discredit the author.

Another line of attacks waged broader accusations into the authenticity of the diary itself, sometimes even calling the very details of its production into question. One of the more commonly discussed points of contention regarding "authenticity" is tied to a diary entry from February 13, 2020, where Fang Fang describes a photograph of a pile of abandoned cellphones at a crematorium, after their owners had been cremated. Here is the passage from *Wuhan Diary*:

> Even more heartbreaking was a photo that a doctor friend texted me. Seeing that image suddenly brought back all the sadness that has been surrounding me these past several days. The picture was of a pile of cellphones piled up

---

[5] Fang Fang. *Wuhan Diary: Dispatches from a Quarantined City*. New York: HarperVia, 2020. Pg. 103.

on the floor of a funeral home; the owners of those phones had already been reduced to ash. No words.[6]

It is a heartbreaking scene that Fang Fang here describes; it is also hard to imagine that this short passage would unleash a wellspring of controversy, triggering more than a year of constant allegations and attacks. Fang Fang's critics accused her of peddling lies and claimed the original February 13 blog post appeared with a doctored photograph; Fang Fang forcefully rejected the validity of these attacks, again responding in her diary:

> I'm in a really terrible mood today. Sometime during the early a.m. hours I discovered that there was someone on Weibo who goes by the name "Xiang Ligang from CCTIME.COM" who ran a photo of cellphones for sale at a secondhand market alongside one of my posts that mentioned cellphones discarded next to a crematorium. He then sent out a message claiming that I was the one who uploaded the photo and accused me of spreading online rumors! My diary posts are always pure text and I never upload accompanying photos. One reader posted a comment directed at Mr. Xiang to point this out, but he didn't respond.[7]

Then on March 20, Fang Fang addressed the issues of the cellphones again, this time in response to an online attack by Peking University Professor Zhang Yiwu 張頤武. Fang Fang quotes a long passage from Zhang's post before offering an extended response:

> As for that photograph, I have already explained that in great detail in an earlier post. So it is a real shame that Professor Zhang seems to have never taken the time to read what I wrote. Actually, Professor Zhang should really come out to Wuhan to understand the true situation firsthand: Then he would understand things like just how many people died each day, how the dead bodies were transported from the hospitals to the crematoriums, what happened to the personal articles of the deceased after they died, what kind of situation the hospitals and crematoriums were in, why lithium batteries cannot be burned, what kind of sterilization methods are being used, and why so many crematoriums all over the country have been supporting Wuhan. But I will have to stop here. For Professor Zhang and others who are willing to understand what is happening, all the information is here; if you don't want to see the truth, that is your choice. I'm sure that one day

[6] Ibid. Pg. 86.
[7] Ibid. Pg. 95.

everyone will see that photograph; but it won't be from me, it needs to come from the person who took that photo. I really recommend that Professor Zhang visit Wuhan so that he can conduct his own firsthand investigation; of course, I should add that all these things occurred during the early stages of the outbreak, not later and not now. I think it would be more in keeping with Peking University's standards if Professor Zhang first took some time to understand the true situation before rushing to make categorical conclusions. I'm sure that will also make the parents of the students he teaches feel much more at ease.[8]

Here was Fang Fang, writing under quarantine in Wuhan amid an unprecedented outbreak as Zhang Yiwu sits more than 700 miles away in Beijing, obsessively posting about a photo of cellphones Fang Fang had briefly mentioned a month earlier. For the trolls attacking Fang Fang, the "mystery of the abandoned cellphones" would be transformed into a salacious cliffhanger fueling a full year of reports, articles, allegations, and attacks. The popular leftist portal Diba 帝吧 widely disseminated a series of political cartoons depicting the origin story of the photo. In this iteration, a scheming, rectangular-headed Fang Fang sneaks a photo of a pile of used cellphones being sold by a street squatter and tries to pass the image off as cellphones of deceased COVID patients. In mid-September even the Communist Youth League weighed in on the cellphone photo controversy. The author of the Chinese blog "American Diary" uploaded a scathing entry about the cellphones on September 21, 2020, and thousands of individual users posted a seemingly endless flood of demands to "show us the cellphone phone!", "what about the photo of the abandoned cellphones?", "how do you explain the cellphone phone?". A video produced by Insight (Mingbian 明辨) listing the Top Ten Internet Hoaxes Young People Are Following of 2019–2020 even listed the cellphone photo as entry number eight. (In the video the "hoax" is that the photo posted online was a fake, which it was; however here it is claimed that Fang Fang intentionally posted the fake photo, an argument which is then used here discredit Fang Fang's entire narrative.) Eventually the story about the abandoned cellphones would be reduced to a meme to attack the United States, with numerous Weibo posts referring to "500,000 abandoned American cellphones," referring to the COVID-19 death toll in the United States at that time. More than 18 months after Fang Fang

---

[8] Ibid. Pg. 324.

published that entry—posts about the now infamous "abandoned cell-phones" continued to appear on Chinese social media as a means of attacking the authenticity of *Wuhan Diary* and attacking the United States.

One wonders, of all the content posted in the diary which spanned 60 entries and more than 140,000 Chinese characters in length (400 pages of content in English translation), why did the trolls repeatedly revisit the abandoned cellphones? I think it has something to do with the primacy of images and the way in which photographs seem to say something different about our notions of truth telling than words. This is tied to longstanding notions of "photographic evidence" which are intimately linked to how we approach the act of witnessing. Fang Fang had already been under attack by the ultra-leftists for not being an "authentic witness" to the outbreak (i.e., she was not a doctor or a frontline worker). Fang Fang powerfully countered in her diary when she wrote:

> I read an essay today that said Fang Fang shouldn't be hiding out at home writing her diary based on gossip she hears; she should get out there in the field where everything is happening! How can I even respond to that? It isn't a question of wanting to get out there in the field; I'm living in the field! The entire city of Wuhan is where this is happening! I am one of the nine million victims of this epidemic. My neighbors, classmates, coworkers are all locked down here in Wuhan; we all are. When they go online and share their experiences and what they have witnessed, why shouldn't I be documenting all of that? Don't tell me that only the sites where these doctors, police officers, and public service people are working qualify as "the field"! I'm here in the field recording what I hear and see, but if you insist on calling that gossip, there is nothing I can say; do as you wish.[9]

But, somehow, the photograph of abandoned cellphones or rather the *absence* of this image became transformed into a metaphor. The fact that the basic narrative of events surrounding the photo was messy and hard to follow probably worked to the benefit of the trolls. The timeline ran something like this: Fang Fang briefly described a photo of abandoned cellphones that she had seen, someone online uploaded a doctored photo, trolls later claimed Fang Fang was responsible for that fake photo, Fang Fang denied these allegations, trolls then demanded Fang upload "the real" photograph that she had initially described, Fang Fang refused since

---

[9] Fang Fang. *Wuhan Diary: Dispatches from a Quarantined City.* New York: HarperVia, 2020, pg. 180.

it was not hers to share, etc. Average netizens in China were not privy to the entire story which allowed trolls to transform it into a black-and-white metaphor or symbol of manufactured truth. Their argument was simple: Fang Fang was uploading fake photos online to make China look bad and capitalize on tragedy. This metaphor of the photo wielded a power beyond its presence or rather, absence. It would stand in for, and eventually harness, months of allegations about doctored truth claims, false accounts, an absence of witnessing, and a lack of firsthand evidence, all of which would be crystalized through the "image" of an imaginary photograph.

Allegations that Fang Fang's diary contained falsehoods became so exaggerated that numerous public figures began to accuse the book of being a work of fiction, including former Taiwan legislator Chiu Yi 邱毅, who claimed in a television interview that later went viral online in China, "Fang Fang's Diary is not a work of reportage literature, it is basically just a work of fiction—an entirely fabricated novel."[10] In an even more unexpected turn, challenges to the authenticity of the book even came in the form of allegations that *Wuhan Diary* was actually a work of manufactured propaganda, produced by the United States (with Fang Fang as a puppet figurehead) in order to attack China. It did not take long for these more aggressive attacks on the authenticity of the diary to begin to slip into the realm of conspiracy theory. As Slavoj Žižek observed in his discussion of the outbreak in Wuhan, the control of information is directly linked to the production of conspiracy theories, "The chief argument against the idea that the state has to control rumors to prevent panic is that this control itself spreads distrust and thus creates even more conspiracy theories."[11]

The pervasive nature of the attacks, criticism, and general debate surrounding *Wuhan Diary* during this period took on a number of different forms. Historian Wu Rui 吳銳 provided a detailed overview of the myriad allegations that sprung up against Fang Fang:

> The Wuhan lockdown was lifted on April 8, 2020. As soon as people learned that Fang Fang's diary was being translated into foreign languages for pub-

---

[10] A short 1:35 video featuring Chiu Yi admonishing Fang Fang as a "third-rate writer," accusing her of being manipulated by the United States, and claiming the diary was purely fictionalized was widely disseminated on Chinese social media during April of 2020 by influential platforms like Observer Network and thousands of individual Weibo users. https://3g.163.com/v/video/VAA28K6EJ.html.

[11] Zizek, Slavoj. *Pandemic!: COVID-19 Shakes the World*. New York: Polity Press, 2020. Pg. 10.

lication abroad, the attacks against Fang Fang reached their climax. Many of Fang Fang's "fans" overnight turned into her "detractors." There were numerous crimes that Fang Fang was accused of online, some of which included being a member of the "American Fifth Column (美國第五縱隊)," being an "anti-China bullet," "passing the knife [to America in order to harm China] (遞刀子)," "one who leads the enemies in to invade (帶路黨)," "sinking the ship by driving it into a wall (撞牆沈船)," "selling out the nation and the people (賣國賣人民)," "bring pain to one's own people and gladdening the enemy (親痛仇快)," and "providing weapons to anti-China forces (為反中力量添磚加瓦)." The single most important line was the "passing the knife theory" (遞刀論), which argued that it didn't matter what [Fang Fang] said within China, but by no means should these negative views be promoted outside of China. By exposing the negative side of the COVID-19 outbreak to the world, she was shaming and humiliating the nation and becoming the "knife" that external forces would use to harm China. In their eyes, this was a fundamental betrayal of China's national interests, the actions of a national traitor that had now identified her as the worst scum of the Chinese people.[12]

Wu Rui captures the conspiratorial nature of so many of the attacks as well as the ways in which the discourse was laden with rhetorical labels and fueled by nationalist sentiment. The fact that news of the international publication of the diary broke on the very day that the 76-day lockdown in Wuhan was lifted only further exacerbated the attacks.

Many of these theories revolved around the origin of the virus, the US-China trade war, and the issues of reparations: three topics which *Wuhan Diary* never directly engaged with, yet somehow got pulled into. Allegations that the diary was attempting to weigh in on "the origin" of the novel coronavirus began with the controversy surrounding the early subtitle of my translation, which was discussed earlier. Although the initial working subtitle only had a shelf life of roughly one week, allegations that Fang Fang, HarperVia, and I were willfully positioning the book as an attempt to pinpoint the "origin" of COVID-19 would persist for more than two years. These allegations were, of course, tied to broader conspiracy theory narratives that were fed by the US-China trade war, increasing diplomatic tension between the two countries, and growing cries from none other than Donald Trump to hold China accountable

[12] Wu Rui 吳銳. Twentieth Century Chinese Historiography and Historians (二十世紀史學與史學家). Taipei: Tonson Publications, 2021. Pg. 764.

"for unleashing" what he deemed "the China virus."[13] The role of US political rhetoric attacking China in fanning the flames of the Chinese disinformation campaign that would ensue should not be underestimated. "A CNN KFile review of Trump's public statements identified at least 12 occasions in which the President praised or projected confidence about China's response to coronavirus"[14] during the early phase of the outbreak, using words like "extremely capable" and Xi Jinping's "doing a very good job with a very, very tough situation" to describe efforts undertaken to contain the outbreak. However, in mid-March the tenor of Trump's statements underwent a radical shift. March 16, 2020, was the first time he used the term "Chinese Virus" in a tweet, which not only went viral but began to generate hashtags and inspire other racially inflected speech.[15] On March 19, 2020, Trump declared "the world is going to pay a very big price for what they [China] did."[16] It didn't take long for other members of the regime to start echoing and amplifying political messages critical of China. On May 3, 2020, Secretary of State Mike Pompeo told ABC's "This Week with George Stephanopoulos" that there was "enormous evidence" that the coronavirus originated in the Wuhan Institute of Virology, a statement not confirmed by heath officials.[17] These criticisms were not relegated to the Republican Party, even then Democratic Presidential candidate Joe Biden began to make hawkish rhetoric about China a major part of his political campaign

[13] Donald Trump has made numerous comments like this throughout 2020; here I am referencing his address to the United Nations on September 22, which was widely reported in the international media, including Rick Gladstone, "Trump Demands U.N. Hold China to Account for Coronavirus Pandemic" New York Times, Dept. 22, 2020. https://www. nytimes.com/2020/09/22/world/americas/UN-Trump-Xi-China-coronavirus.html.

[14] Nathan McDermott and Andrew Kaczynski. "Trump Repeatedly Praised China's Response to Coronavirus in February" CC, March 25, 2020.

[15] Dr. Mishal Reja. "Trump's 'Chinese Virus' tweet helped lead to rise in racist anti-Asian Twitter content: Study" ABC News. March 18, 2021. https://abcnews.go.com/Health/trumps-chinese-virus-tweet-helped-lead-rise-racist/story?id=76530148

[16] Dan Mangan. "Trump blames China for coronavirus pandemic: 'The world is paying a very big price for what they did'" CNBC March 19, 2020. https://www.cnbc.com/2020/03/19/coronavirus-outbreak-trump-blames-china-for-virus-again.html

[17] Deb Riechmann and Zeke Miller. "Trump's anti-China rhetoric aimed at boosting US leverage" AP May 4, 2020. https://apnews.com/article/virus-outbreak-donald-trump-us-news-ap-top-news-politics-e981e084208ec5dc3c93d9e5b5ae234a

messaging in April of 2020.[18] The deluge of attacks that would rain down upon *Wuhan Diary* need to be looked at within the context of the sudden rise of US political attacks, negative messaging, and "blame game" rhetoric concerning China. This global political context is crucial for a more nuanced understanding of the ideological fuel that became one of the pre-conditions for the ensuing attacks; it also helps illustrate another facet of why the disinformation campaign against Fang Fang's book was indeed "transpacific," born, in part, by the anti-China rhetoric that came to a crescendo in the United States between March and April of 2020.

Of course, when the translation commenced on February 25, 2020, and when HarperVia purchased North American rights to *Wuhan Diary* in early March, topics like "blaming China" for unleashing COVID-19 or "exacting reparations" from China did not exist; yet the book's critics in China insisted the entire production of the book had been a well-conceived plot on the part of the Americans. The rhetoric surrounding "American imperialist conspiracies" also harkened back to the worn-out tropes left-over from the Korean War; it is no coincidence that the Chinese film industry also began production on a new litter of "Resist-America Aid North Korea" war films in 2020.

Beginning on April 8, articles, posts, and messages on Weibo and other platforms began to unleash a grab-bag of wild and sometimes self-contradictory accusations: Fang Fang was an agent for the Nationalist regime in Taiwan, I was a CIA agent, the book was actually translated by a crack team of CIA translators working around the clock, I was the "real" author and Fang Fang was translating my fabricated lies into Chinese to deceive local readers, and on the tales went. In December 2020 there was even a wave of conspiracy theories circulating online in China that claimed *Wuhan Diary* was secretly backed by the American branch of the Freemasonry Society![19] But by far, the single most widely

---

[18] See, for instance, Peter Beinart's article in *The Atlantic,* "The Utter Futility of Biden's China Rhetoric" April 20, 2020. https://www.theatlantic.com/ideas/archive/2020/04/futility-bidens-china-hawkery/610285/.

[19] For a video discussing and dispelling this allegation, see the video posted by Lao Yang Daochushuo 老楊到處說 entitled "Is Fang Fang a Member of the Freemasons!?" ("Fang Fang shi Gongjihuiyuan!?" 方方是共濟會員!?) to YouTube on December 2, 2020: https://www.youtube.com/watch?v=usc8wShVEuw.

circulated and impactful conspiracy theory involved Fang Fang's very decision to publish *Wuhan Diary* abroad (with the United States and Germany singled out). In the eyes of the ultra-nationalists waging these attacks, this was not a simple case of *jiachou buke waiyang* 家醜不可外揚, the old Chinese idiom "one should never air disgraceful family affairs in public"; although there was certainly some dimension of that, it, instead, amounted to nothing less than an act of treason. Yet here we do see the alignment of the feudal, patriarchal fixation of *jiachou buke waiyang* running parallel to nationalist pride, simultaneously engaging with both old leftists from the Cultural Revolution generation and the new post-1990s "Little Pink" leftists. It was alleged that Fang Fang was handing a sharp knife over to the United States, which they, in turn, would use to humiliate, punish, and hurt China. It was simultaneously alleged that the publication of *Wuhan Diary* would further enflame racial tension in the United States, leading to increased cases of violence against Chinese-Americans and Asian-Americans, who would be targeted and blamed. Seeing the onslaught of conspiracy theories play out and evolve day by day was like entering a strange topsy-turvy universe where truth itself was being willfully inverted and replaced by a revolving sideshow of tall takes and stories of the fantastic. This flood of disinformation is, of course, all part of a larger strategy of distraction. In this case, repeated criticisms and attacks focusing on small details (like the photo of cellphones) and the fabrications of lies and rumors are part of a campaign to distract from larger issues such as Fang Fang's calls for accountability and her sobering revelations about the violent nature of Chinese web culture. Looked at as a continuum, over the course of the many months of prolonged attacks, the crucial turning point in the attempt to purge Fang Fang was news of the English and German translation of the book; this was the moment that allowed the old specters of xenophobia and revanchism to suddenly reappear.

The abrupt shift in tone amongst the Chinese media regarding Fang Fang was so radical that *China Law Review* (*Zhongguo falu pinglun* 中國法律評論) even published a comprehensive study of the sudden change in attitude towards the diary amongst different groups. Led by a team of four researchers from the Tsinghua University School of Law and based on a focus group consisting of 109 students, the study found (as summarized by Fedtke, Ibahrine, and Wang): "In terms of their attitude toward the diary, 38 (34.86%) say that they are against the diary, 16.51% say that they changed their attitude from supportive to against, 20.18% say that they support the diary, 26.61% say that they do not care, only 2 students (1.83%) say that they changed from against to support."[20] According to the survey, 65 people (approximately 60% of the participants) strongly agreed or somewhat agreed with the statement that speech should be subjugated to larger national interests during exceptional times (26% disagreed or strongly disagreed, while 14% were unsure). Besides the findings, the very existence of such a research project, which was published on April 18, 2020, just ten days after the uproar over the foreign publication of *Wuhan Diary* erupted, also speaks to how powerfully the controversy had been reverberating through Chinese society at that time.

Running in unison with these larger conspiratorial theories as described by Wu Rui and other claims about the alleged US political backing for the book was a parallel campaign of personal attacks. Some of them were predictable: Fang Fang was just a petty opportunist, aimed at using her diary to leverage fame and wealth. In actuality, as soon as Fang Fang decided to publish *Wuhan Diary* abroad she made the decision to donate all of her profits to the families of frontline medical workers who had died during the initial coronavirus outbreak in Wuhan. In October of 2020 she donated more than $180,000 USD to family members of deceased medical workers via the Henghui Charity Foundation 恆輝兒童公益基金會. Throughout 2020 the trolls paid no heed to the fact that Fang Fang had committed to donate her proceeds to charity. Instead they painted her as a greedy profiteer. (One popular accusation widely shared on Chinese social media was that Fang Fang was paid 12 million US dollars in royalties for writing her diary!)[21] They launched their own series of official complaints and slanderous "investigations" into Fang Fang's finances, property holdings, and history of international travel, attempting to paint her as someone swimming in elitist entitlement. These came in the form of thousands of online posts as well as numerous professionally produced

[20] For the original report, see Chen, Xinyu; Zhuo, Zenghua; Xu, Yichen; and Wu, Zhihang (2020), Report of a Survey on Fang Fang Diary ('Fang Fang Riji wenjuan Diaocha Yanjiu Baogao'方方日記問卷調查研究報告), China Law Review (Zhongguo Falu Pinglun 中國法律評論), available at https://wemp.app/posts/299b0cb7-41b3-4c5b-9f32-e06e145ac9ca. A short English-language summary of the major findings of the survey can also be found in Jana Fedtke, Mohammed Ibahrine, and Yuting Wang. "Corona crisis chronicle: Fang Fang's *Wuhan Diary* (2020) as an act of sousveillance" *Online Information Review* February 23, 2021. Pg. 805. https://www.emerald.com/insight/1468-4527.htm.
[21] One such article was published on May 1, 2020, by Chinese Legal Aid Network entitled "Expose on Fang Fang: She Made 12 Million US Dollars, She Bragged About it Online and Her Friends Congratulated Her With Flowers" (方方現狀爆光，靠出版日記怒賺1200萬美金，發文炫耀有人送花) http://m.cnflyz.org/fyyy/20200501/25594.html.

"investigative report" style videos.[22] Many of these accusations, attacks, and amateur "investigations" could be identified as a "human-flesh search," which has been defined as a way in which "netizens use their internet search skills to hunt for information aimed to expose the alleged misdemeanors of individuals ranging from animal abusers to party officials suspected of corruption. Smacking of internet vigilantism, human-flesh search resembles a collective quest for truth or social justice."[23] In this case, however, the human-flesh search was employed not in the spirit of truth, but in order to disseminate misinformation and carry out intimidation. Like the earlier discussed photo of abandoned cellphones, another detail was culled from Fang Fang's diary to "prove" her elitist manipulation of the system: a description of how Fang Fang asked a policeman she knew for help to escort her niece to the airport. At the time, Wuhan was completely locked down, taxis and public transportation were not running, and her niece, a Singapore citizen, was trying to get to the airport to board a flight chartered by the Singapore government to evacuate their citizens. Like the cellphone incident, this too would get rehashed ad nauseam for months to come, all cited as further evidence of Fang Fang's privilege and so-called crimes. After completely ignoring the fact that Fang Fang has donated proceeds from her book to charity, in early 2021 trolls began to allege that Fang Fang never actually donated any of the money she had promised. When official charity donation receipts were finally made public, trolls went so far as to attack the Henghui Charity Foundation.

Collectively, these attacks can be seen as a concerted attempt to methodically tear down the "myth" of Fang Fang. Over the course of her serialized posts, Fang Fang had built up a loyal and robust readership, her personal style had made her readers feel as if they knew her, and millions of them waited up each night to read her next diary installment. According to Guobin Yang, "each diary entry was a social media sensation."[24] And,

---

[22] For instance, this report produced by "Voice of the Dragon" (Long zhi sheng 龍之聲) was posted to YouTube on April 29, 2020, entitled: "Headline News Today! They Have Dug Out the Dirt! There is a Huge Secret Lurking Within Fang Fang's Villa That No One Can Imagine! The Shocking Scandal is Now Exposed for All to See!" ("Jinri toutiao! Zhongyu chachulai le! Fang Fang bieshu laowu ancang yizhuang jingtian da mimi, chaochu le suoyouren xiangxiang! Jingtianheimu baoguang, dabaiyutianxia!" 今日頭條！終於查出來了！方方別墅老屋暗藏一樁驚天動地的秘密，超出了所有人想像！驚天黑幕爆光大白於天下！) https://www.youtube.com/watch?v=87EKrim11DI.
[23] Guobin Yang. *The Wuhan Lockdown*. New York: Columbia University Press: 2021. Pg. 23.
[24] Guobin Yang. *The Wuhan Lockdown*. New York: Columbia University Press, 2021. Pg. 83.

in the words of Kevin Robins, "*Wuhan Diary* was actually a "live" event, released in daily installments through various Chinese social media platforms…It was an epic of improvisation. And rather than an author, Fang Fang might be best thought of as a kind of hybrid between a compiler and a conductor."[25] The broad base of her support, in part, explains the ruthless and multifaceted approach employed to tear her down. A simplistic attack on just one aspect of *Wuhan Diary* could never compete with the grassroots support she had been receiving from millions of Chinese readers all over the world; instead a more sophisticated approach was needed. That approach necessitated not just an attack on the diary, but also personal attacks on Fang Fang herself; what transpired was no less than an act of cyber-character assassination. The trolls were waging an ideological war meant to slander and defame her, aiming much of their messaging towards disenfranchised internet users in lower-income brackets without advanced education—hence the attention placed on exposing Fang Fang's so-called wealth and privilege. During the early COVID-19 outbreak when many locations in China were locked down and people were unable to work, these unemployed workers were angry, frustrated, and suffering from real economic hardships; highlighting Fang Fang's so-called entitlement and traitorous actions was a way of directing their anger towards a tangible target that represented privilege and exploitation. It was also a sophisticated attempt to harness and manipulate longstanding feelings of class difference and disenfranchisement in the ideological warfare being waged against *Wuhan Diary*. If, over those few short weeks from late February through early April, Fang Fang had gone from a fairly well-known writer to one of the most popular and talked-about figures in China, a hero to millions of readers, this campaign was intent on, one rumor at a time, dismantling that myth. Turning again to Guobin Yang:

> More than just a target, Fang Fang was weaponized. Attacking her was a means of shutting down all criticisms of the party authorities. Who would dare speak up again if they witnessed the endless and random verbal violence against Fang Fang? Quite a few diarists mentioned that after Fang Fang's diary became a national controversy, they stopped sharing personal views about it on WeChat for fear of alienating friends and family.[26]

---

[25] Kevin Robins. "The Great City is Fragile: Fang Fang's *Wuhan Diary.*" *Cultural Politics*, Volume 17, Issue 1. Duke University Press, 2021. Pg. 73.
[26] Guobin Yang. *The Wuhan Lockdown.* New York: Columbia University Press, 2021. Pg. 150.

Fang Fang responded in depth to the multitude of attacks, first in her diary itself, in shorter Weibo posts, through in-depth interviews with official mainstream news outlets, and, most substantially, in a series of long-form essays posted on Weibo under the title "About" ("Guanyu" 關於) which she began posting immediately after completing the 60-day diary. However, the nature of the attacks remained difficult to counter due to the very means by which they are waged and the later removal of many of Fang Fang's own interviews and articles from the internet.

The attacks became so pervasive that much of the global media's coverage of *Wuhan Diary* began to focus more on the persecution of Fang Fang and the various threats she received than the book itself. While the trolls were attacking Fang Fang for "selling out China to the world," those very attacks became the primary fuel that was helping make the book into a global phenomenon. In other words, while the trolls criticized Fang Fang for allegedly sharing China's dirty secrets to the world, it was in fact their very attacks that were constantly bringing even more global attention to the book. In the process, their actions were revealing an even more scathing inditement—not about COVID-19—but about how disinformation campaigns in China function. It is therefore disingenuous for detractors of the book to criticize Fang Fang for *chongyang meiwai* 崇洋媚外 (worshipping the foreign and pandering to Westerners) or *jiachou buke waiyang* (washing dirty laundry in public) when their attacks and posts are, in fact, an essential part of the symbiotic relationship between global and Chinese media. Throughout 2020, each and every time any major Western media outlet—*The New York Times, The Los Angeles Times*, BBC, *The London Times, The Economist*, etc.—published any coverage about Fang Fang, those articles immediately (often within the span of a few hours) became fodder for more troll attacks. And thus the cycle perpetuated itself.

So how were the attacks waged? I describe the attacks against *Wuhan Diary* as a campaign because it was not a simplistic case of a group of internet trolls writing nasty comments online; this was something much more complex and sophisticated operation that played out simultaneously on multiple levels. In order to sway public opinion that had been overwhelmingly supportive of Fang Fang and effectively "change the conversation," the cyber campaign reached deep into its toolbox, alternately employing (1) social media attacks, (2) death threats, (3) disinformation campaign/employment of "fake news," (4) a witch hunt aimed at silencing stories and individuals defending Fang Fang, (5) employment of "pop culture" to discredit and mock Fang Fang, (6) pressure to suppress the publication of *Wuhan Diary*, and (7) an inundation of parallel "official narratives" to offset the version of events presented in Fang Fang's diary. There was a clear sense of orchestration in the way in which all of these different tactics were simultaneously employed.

One of the earliest and most visible hallmarks of the campaign was a sharp spike in social media posts attacking Fang Fang and her diary. The vast majority of these attacks were posted on Weibo, which became the primary battleground for the ideological warfare being waged against *Wuhan Diary*. They came in the form of thousands of attacks uploaded to the comments sections of Fang Fang's diary entries and articles about the diary as well as original posts launching more directed attacks upon the blog. Early on, many of the accounts were the same individuals and units that had come after *Soft Burial* three years earlier and, eventually, a core group of antagonists emerged. Some of the more influential platforms and individuals targeting Fang Fang included Xiang Ligang of CCTIME. COM 項立剛, Peking University Professor Zhang Yiwu, Cartoonist Yam Bear Six 地瓜熊老六, vlogger and political commentator Sima Nan 司馬南, the website Observer Network 觀察者網, and the website Red Culture 紅色文化網, which had actually published the original three essays attacking *Soft Burial* back in 2017. Many of these influential Weibo users can be characterized as "political influencers" and they were posting repeatedly about *Wuhan Diary*. For instance, Zhang Yiwu first posted about *Wuhan Diary* on March 21 to attack the infamous "photo of abandoned cellphones," and, over the course of the next seven months, he would go on to upload more than 70 posts, including numerous long-form essays, attacking the diary. On Weibo each of these accounts has massive numbers of followers making their reach and influence extremely potent.[27] These "leftist" VIP users also receive preferential treatment by various platforms in terms of how their posts are processed, even allowing them to upload content with "sensitive keywords" which would normally be banned if posted by regular users. As former Weibo employee Eric Liu noted in an interview:

[27] For instance, as of October 9, 2020, Yam Bear Six had over six million followers, Zhang Yiwu over eight million followers, and Xiang Ligang over one million followers.

All of China's media platforms give special treatment to patriotic social media users, which are referred to as "positive energy VIPs"; they include accounts by professionals like Sima Nan as well as the individual accounts of members of the net police, cadres from the Ministry of Propaganda, and official accounts of the Communist Youth League….The measuring stick when it comes to censorship that is applied to these users is shockingly different from that of your average Weibo users. When conducting searches for "sensitive terms" you discover that these (positive energy VIP users) are the only ones who can actually post anything (employing those terms).[28]

Reviews of the diary published overseas in outlets like *The New York Times*, *The New Yorker*, and *The New York Review of Books* were attacked on Weibo within hours of publication; even reviews that were not at all controversial were framed through an anti-American perspective and passages were excerpted and translated through an ideologically skewed lens. The international reviews fed the activity of the Chinese trolls and the broad influence of the VIP Weibo accounts leading the charge enabled the campaign against Fang Fang to quickly recruit and mobilize millions of internet users who, in turn, would post their own attacks, exponentially increasing online activity on the topic.

As I translated *Wuhan Diary*, from February 25 through mid-April, I would try to stay focused on the task at hand, yet all the while I was of course keenly aware of the attacks being waged. I would occasionally see them pop up on my Weibo feed, Fang Fang and friends would text me about them, and, of course, they gradually crept into the diary proper, becoming one of the main narrative threads towards the end of the 60-day run. I tried to remain sensitive to the impact and ramifications of the attacks (especially for Fang Fang), while, at the same time, I knew there was no way I could fully comprehend what she must have been experiencing. But then, in early April as pre-sales information about *Wuhan Diary* appeared on Amazon.com (at that point there had still not even been an official press release from HarperVia announcing publication), the trolls came for me. The first message I received was a text from a friend on the morning of April 7 (April 8 in China) warning me not to check my Weibo account. I did anyway, and, when I did log on, this is what I saw:

---

[28] Interview with Eric Liu, May 11, 2021.

April 8, 2020 23:57	Please never ever come back to China! The Chinese people do not welcome you!
April 8, 2020 23:44	*Your family will live in the hell forever and never get peace*
April 8, 2020 23:42	*Your son will die in three days*
April 8, 2020 23:36	Hello CIA, Goodbye CIA
April 8, 2020 23:31	*Spreading fake news in China. You and your mate Fang Fang are completely not welcome in China.*
April 8, 2020 23:30	*Fu*k U!!!*
April 8, 2020 23:29	The waters are deep, careful not to drown.
April 8, 2020 23:21	*Fuck you white pig*
April 8, 2020 23:18	*You mother fucker*
April 8, 2020 23:14	The CIA created departments of East Asian Languages with the sole intention of carrying out subversion!
April 8, 2020 23:06	Have you gotten COVID-19 yet? It will be there soon, you deserve your herd immunity!
April 8, 2020 23:06	*Fuck off*
April 8, 2020 19:55	*Fuck your mum*
April 8, 2020 19:48	*I heard you recreate the liar diary. So funny the fake diary can be part of record of the islation of a hero city*
April 8, 2020 19:38	*And hope your family being infected by AMERICAN VIRUS*

April 8,	*American liar. Check how many poor American ppl died because of your*
2020	*government stupidity. I believe your American diary will be much more colorful*
19:32	*and PAINFUL! Shame on you LIAR! Your Jesus will not will the cheater like you!*
April 8,	*Shame on you*
2020	
19:31	

Sample of some of the messages posted to my Weibo account on April 8, 2020. Text in italics originally appeared in English. Other text is translated from Chinese.

These were just a fraction of the messages posted as part of the comments thread of a Weibo post that had been originally uploaded on February 1, 2020. The post had actually been, ironically enough, an announcement for the roundtable forum on COVID-19 that I had co-organized at UCLA. Since it had been my most recent post, that is where there attacks initially gravitated. Within just a few hours there were 300 comments, by the next day there would be 600; over the course of the next few weeks there would be more than 4482 comments uploaded to the message threads on various posts on my Weibo account and the message threads containing the attacks would be viewed more than 6 million times. Many of the comments and messages came from fake accounts with user names like "Fang Fang Goes to Jail" (方方進監獄了) or "America is a Complete Failure" (美國徹底失敗吧), indicating they had been specifically created in order to attack *Wuhan Diary*. Typical comments included:

The quarantine was just lifted today in Wuhan and Grandma Fang Fang's Diary has already been published in English and German. Wow, the CIA really moves at light speed! If the American government could act as quickly in battling the coronavirus America would never suffer from so many deaths and infections!

You Americans are part of a failed nation and you still manage to keep all your attention focused on others! The CIA is the biggest terrorist organization in the world; they specialize in training poisonous sewer rats like you. It is disgusting. [middle finger emoji]

I hope you will have the opportunity to write a diary about your own dirty country!

Wuhan Diary is FAKE STORY! FAKE DAIRY! Go hell! (sic.)

You are a liar just the same as FF is! Shame on you both!

You should write an "American Diary"! Write about how Trump has neglected the lives of the American people! Do you dare? All you do is spread rumors in China! You Coward! [three thumbs down emojis]

Fang Fang's is bad to the bone; now that she has been dragged through the mud she has thrown Mr. Berry to the wolves…This white guy is real idiot. He carried her sedan chair for her and, now that he has outlived his usefulness, she has abandoned him and thrown him away. It is pathetic, sad and infuriating!

The translator of a liar is also a liar. Shame on you!

Mr. Berry, perhaps you don't realize it, but you have made a lot of mistakes by translating *Fang Fang's Diary*. Your translation has left many Chinese feeling unhappy with you. We even feel that your translation has helped some Americans to insult China. Moreover, your translation seems to carry with it a certain prejudice in the way in which you use an American perspective to look at Chinese issues. This is wrong. I hope that if you ever come back to China you take the time to look around some provincial small towns to understand things.

The Chinese language has been insulted by your very use of the language, all because of you.

American liar. Check how many poor American ppl died because of your government stupidity. I believe your America Diary will be much more colorful and PAINFUL! Shame on you LIAR! Your Jesus will not will the cheater like you! (sic.)

Mr. Berry, you have successfully translated a book that most Chinese people deem to be a putrid book and now you have given us a putrid translation. That means that you are responsible! Because of this a lot of Chinese are cursing you; you will not get an apology from me, nor an ounce of compassion. Your decision was perhaps steeped in malicious intentions or perhaps it was due to your own oversight; but it was *your* decision and now you must face the consequences. We Chinese are able to make a clear distinction between right and wrong.

Fangfang's diary is part of your ANTI-CHINA INDUSTRY, congratulations.

Your family will live in the hell forever and never get peace

Have you contracted COVID-19 yet? It's coming soon; you deserve to have your herd immunity.

You translated it as she wrote it? Don't you mean you co-wrote it and later translated it?

The true author of *Wuhan Diary* has been revealed to be Michael Berry; Fang Fang is the translator.

Michael Berry is gone; but he didn't leave in peace; his body was left in the morgue for three days. As they were cremating his body, he suddenly came back to life screaming "I'm not dead!" They had to tie him down with steel cuffs in order to complete the cremation. Once his remains were loaded into the hearse, the car flipped over, spreading his ashes all over the ground. The wind blew most of his ashes away and just as they were about to sweep them up, a watering car drove by. As it sprayed water all over the street and, over the loudspeaker, the announcement came: "Today is a great day, the family members all stayed strong and nobody cried; one of them even laughed!" Later they buried the gentleman but as soon as they left lightning struck, splitting his tombstone in half.[29]

The quotes above are but a small sampling of the thousands of comments and attacks posted on my Weibo page, which are, in turn, but a tiny fraction of the number of attacks that Fang Fang has received. While posts criticizing me continued to appear online for more than two years, the vast majority of the attacks were concentrated between April and June of 2020; Fang Fang on the other hand has been subjected to a much more intense and protracted online campaign. Once I became targeted, I suddenly found myself with a renewed understanding of what Fang Fang had been going through and the remarkable act of bravery required for her to persevere and continue writing in the face of such vicious attacks. As I pushed through and completed the final pages of the translation amid the onslaught of these posts, I often felt like I was racing down a highway littered with crashes and explosions all around me; it took a great deal of focus to keep my eyes on the road. I can only imagine how Fang Fang managed when the attacks were so much more vicious, often tainted with misogynistic threats of sexual violence, exponential in number, and, of course, with her living in China, the stakes were much higher.

I considered shutting my Weibo account down or closing the comments thread function on my posts; I actually temporarily did take the latter measure, but after a few days I opened it back up again. I thought of Fang Fang and how she had written about the importance of preserving the attacks as a kind of digital museum to attest to this age of absurdity:

A good thing, then, that the internet has a memory, and that memory lasts a long time. And so I think I should preserve the message thread on my Weibo account as an observation point—a living record of this era to preserve for the future. Preserved in the memory of every era are beautiful and moving things right there alongside those painful and sad things. But what usually leaves the deepest impression is always shame. It is particularly important to preserve those shameful acts of this age, as well. This flood of

---

[29] All of these comments were posted in the comments thread to my February 1, 2020, post on Weibo; the majority of the comments above were all posted on April 8, 2020, the day the attacks commenced. https://weibo.com/2500448414/Is82azfPm?filter=hot&root_comment_id=0&type=comment.

collective curses and insults serves as a record of the most humiliating and shameful documents of this era. When people in the future one day look back and read these comments posted in 2020, they will see that, as a virus was spreading in Wuhan, another virus was infecting people's language online and spreading all over my Weibo message board. The spread of the coronavirus led to the unprecedented quarantine of millions of people within this city, while the virus infecting my Weibo account clearly unveiled the true shame of this era.[30]

And so the posts remain. I did, however, go through a decade's worth of my past Weibo posts, systematically removing all photos and videos of my children, which I had occasionally uploaded over the years. Although the target of the attacks was a contemporary diary documenting a public health crisis, the language of the attacks was a historical throwback to the mob mentality that had gripped China during the 1950s; suddenly all of the anti-American rhetoric and conspiracy theories from the past were resurrected and re-employed to purge the translation of a pandemic diary.

There was a deep sense of frustration with the black-and-white way in which the translation was framed as an "anti-Chinese political act," the way in which assumptions were made about my own stance vis-à-vis the original work (again, just because you translate a work by no means you agree with every word published in the original), the way in which critics attributed outright lies and slanderous comments to Fang Fang and me, and especially how *Wuhan Diary* came to be viewed almost exclusively as a text intervening into the ongoing diplomatic tensions between China and the United States. I actually agreed with many of the troll comments criticizing the United States' handling of the coronavirus outbreak, which is in part what drove me to translate the work so quickly! But here my actions were being twisted into a very different political narrative in which I was somehow serving the GOP and Trump regime. I was also surprised by the markedly racist angle that so many of the attacks took on. Some of the most frequently posted curses aimed at me on Weibo included "white nationalist," "racist," "Nazi" (even though I'm Jewish!), and "white pig," which appeared hundreds of times in my message box. There is not much of a silver lining to these attacks, but as a white male living in the wake of the #MeToo movement and Black Lives Matter, I had been reflecting on

---

[30] Fang Fang. *Wuhan Diary: Dispatches from a Quarantined City.* New York: HarperVia, 2020. Pg. 290.

white privilege and systemic racism in America and I tried to take away what lessons I could. At the least, I attempted to use the attacks as way to make myself more sensitive to the struggles of others facing racialized threats and violence on a daily basis. It also spurred me to reflect upon the plight of many generations of Chinese writers and intellectuals who have fallen victim to the politicized attacks and the modern literary inquisition. I thought of writers like Wu Han, author of *Hai Rui Dismissed from Office*, and Lao She, one of China's greatest modern novelists. Both of whom suffered horrendous persecution and eventually died during the Cultural Revolution due to their "literary crimes"—Lao She committed suicide in 1966 and Wu Han died in prison in 1969. I had taught their works and told their stories in the classroom for nearly 20 years; it would be arrogant to think that what I had experienced could come anywhere close to the terrible violence and attacks they faced, but in some sense, it did allow me a small glimpse into what some aspects of those experiences might feel like. I felt I understood them just a little bit better. As best as I could, I tried to take those lessons life presented to me and learn what I could from them, even the ugly ones. Nevertheless, there is no escaping the very real sense of psychological terrorism that such attacks unleash. This, of course, was exacerbated by the second form of personal attacks: death threats.

It is easy to lump threats of bodily harm together with all the other racist and abusive comments posted online, but there is something particularly sinister and nefarious about death threats. While there were numerous death threats that appeared in the comments threads of posts on my Weibo page, the majority of death threats came in the form of private messages sent via Weibo. Most came as short simple messages like "you will die as a dog" or "I want to kill your mother and son"; others were a bit more creative, "You think we are still in the year 1840 and this is the fall of the Great Qing Empire? You ugly white devil, feasting on the flesh of man and drinking human blood, the eighteen realms of hell were created especially for you!" or my favorite: "If you ever set foot in China again I will kill you" followed by a second text ten minutes later, "Sorry, I had too much to drink, I shouldn't have said that." Besides the psychological terrorism mentioned earlier, the numerous threats to bodily injury also serve a potent form of intimidation aimed at silencing victims. While I certainly took the threats seriously, I also knew that being based in Los Angeles and without any immediate family members in China, I was fortunate to have a layer of security; that, however, was not the case for Fang Fang.

   In concert with the anti-Fang Fang social media posts on Chinese platforms like Weibo and WeChat, there was a parallel disinformation campaign being waged through more "official" websites, media portals, and publishing platforms. For instance, the website Red Culture Web, which had published the initial attacks on *Soft Burial* three years earlier, hosted a specially curated portal on its website dedicated to criticizing *Wuhan Diary*. Entitled "A Criticism of Fang Fang's Quarantine Diary," the webpage hosted links to 22 articles attacking Fang Fang. The articles featured titles like "Madame Fang Fang, Please Clear the Feudal Garbage Out of Your Brain!", "During the Quarantine, Fang Fang Abused Her Privilege to Secretly Get Her Niece Out of Wuhan," "How Should Fang Fang Be Dealt With?", and "The Last Thing the Battle Against the Coronavirus Needs are 'Bystanders' Like Fang Fang."[31] And this represents just one of several websites actively involved in attacking *Wuhan Diary*. There were also more official responses, such as a June 10, 2020, article published on China Military, the official news portal of the People's Liberation Army entitled "The Lightspeed Publication of 'Fang Fang's Diary' Will Only Expose the Truth About More Western 'Pot Throwing.'"[32] As David Bandurski of the China Media Project noted, "The suggestion in the article is that unspecified "forces" in Europe and North America wish to use accounts like that of Fang Fang to blacken China's name over the Covid-19 epidemic in order to direct attention away from the worsening situation in their own countries in terms of coronavirus infections and the epidemic response."[33] Other official media outlets like the *Global Times* 環球時報, a daily tabloid newspaper run by the *People's Daily*, also published numerous articles aimed at discrediting Fang Fang, such as "Chinese vigilant on deifying writer Fang Fang amid publication of Wuhan Diary in English" (April 8, 2020) and "'Wuhan Diary' writer escalates online spat, wears out dwindling fans" (April 23, 2020). The editor of the *Global Times*, Hu

---

[31] http://www.hswh.org.cn/htzx/jingji/2020-05-09/25.html

[32] Rao Yufeng 饒玉峰 and Huang Yuqi 黃昱綺. "The Lightspeed Publication of 'Fang Fang's Diary' Will Only Expose the Truth About More Western 'Pot Throwing.'" ("Guangshu chubande FangFang riji, zhineng baolu gengduo xifang 'shuaiguo' de zhenxiang" 光速出版的《方方日記》，只能暴露更多西方 "甩鍋" 的真相) June 10, 2020 on China Military (Zhongguo junwang 中國軍網): http://www.81.cn/jwgd/2020-06/10/content_9832032.htm

[33] David Bandurski. "PLA Site Attacks Bad Domestic Media" June 23, 2020 on China Media Project: https://chinamediaproject.org/2020/06/23/caixin-online-called-anti-china-over-fang-fang-diary-publication/

Xijin 胡錫進, also came out as one of the author's more outspoken critics. Whereas criticisms of the book in February and March were largely spearheaded by individuals and ultra-nationalist websites, when governmental organizations like the PLA and the *Global Times* began to weigh in in early April, it seemed to indicate a clear sign that discourse around *Wuhan Diary* was transforming. Another sign of the changing tide was when Zhang Boli 張伯禮, a physician, an academician of the Chinese Academy of Engineering, and a delegate to the National People's Congress, directly attacked Fang Fang during a May 12, 2020, livestream lecture. Referring to Fang Fang, Zhang claimed: "We have found some people running in the opposite direction, represented by Fang Fang. Some professors and students from universities made improper comments amid the epidemic, exposing their distorted values and twisted souls,"[34] and commenting on the infamous scandal regarding the photograph of abandoned cellphones, Zhang endorsed the rumors that "Fang Fang was trying to send some 'evidence' to anti-China forces so they could attack China through those exaggerated and fabricated stories, but it got a cold reception, as the epidemic situation outside China is now far more chaotic than within China."[35] Fang Fang immediately struck back on Weibo and demanded an apology, but that only led to continued escalation. It was as if the months of attacks and disinformation articles being circulated online were beginning to impact official government interpretations on how the diary should be framed.

Many official media platforms also picked up "chatter" from the trolls circulating on social media and transformed those rumors into "news stories" which provided added validity and attention to what were essentially conspiracy theories. The symbiotic relationship between online internet trolls and official media outlets was repeatedly demonstrated throughout the campaign against Fang Fang. When trolls started claiming *Wuhan Diary* was being weaponized by the West to hurt China, Chinese media outlets quickly picked up the story, and, as the story become more widely disseminated, more trolls came on board. Another example involved conspiracy theories regarding the North American edition's publication date. HarperVia had adjusted the official publication date several times due to

[34] "Some Chinese intellectuals hold distorted values, represented by Fang Fang: academician Zhang Boli" The Global Times. May 14, 2020 (no author byline cited). https://www.globaltimes.cn/content/1188347.shtml
[35] Ibid.

various uncertainties regarding COVID-19, printing schedules, and the translation and editorial schedule. Sometime in April, the date of May 19, 2020, was announced as the publication date for the e-book and audio-book versions of *Wuhan Diary*. Then, in early May, just a few weeks before publication, detractors of the book began spreading rumors that the "anti-China faction" had intentionally selected this date in order to sabotage the "Two Sessions" (兩會, the annual plenary sessions of the People's Congress and the Chinese People's Political Consultative Conference), which had just been announced to take place on May 21, 2020. There was of course no conspiracy. Editors at HarperVia had never heard of the "Two Sessions," the date of which had not even been publicly announced when the May 19 publication date was set. Yet through this mutually rein-forcing relationship between social media rumors and official media out-lets, the conspiracy theory was quickly picked up in official reports and began to circulate widely. One outlet even ran the headline "Publication date of the English edition of Fang Fang's Diary has been moved up, becoming a true bullet." According to the report:

> The English edition of the diary is being released early, setting its target on the "Two Sessions" scheduled to be held between May 21–22 in Beijing. The Two Sessions have always been of the utmost importance to our coun-try which is why these external forces are trying to use the publication of Fang Fang's Diary as a bullet. Who could have imagined that the English edition of Fang Fang's diary would indeed become a bullet that would end up impacting our nation in ways that are difficult to estimate. As we write, the American publisher is working overtime to translate, format, print, and sell Fang Fang's Diary.[36]

Here we can see how the rumors not only triggered numerous official articles, but even led to concerned local officials paying a visit to Fang Fang to discuss these allegations. After the author received pressure to adjust the publication date, the publisher moved the official publication date up a few days to May 15 in order to avoid even the semblance that the diary was somehow intended to interfere with the Two Sessions. But what this example is most illustrative of is how a series of utterly baseless

---

[36] Tietouwa 鐵頭娃. "Publication date of the English edition of Fang Fang's Diary has been moved up, becoming a true bullet." ("Fang Fang yingwenban riji tiqian chuban, zhen chengle yike zidan" 方方英文版日記提前出版，真誠了一顆子彈), May 2, 2020. https://dy.163.com/article/FBK3GTEQ053717V3.html

rumors spread by the book's detractors online were quickly multiplied and amplified to the point that they actually impacted the production schedule of the book.

Beyond the deluge of official articles, there were also a series of academic works published in an attempt to lend academic legitimacy to the attacks. Authored by professors and researchers affiliated with leading academic institutions in China, like Fudan University and Wuhan University, these scholarly contributions included peer-reviewed articles and even full-length monographs, all targeting *Wuhan Diary*. I thought that my translation of Fang Fang's diary was already "lightspeed" but apparently I was no match for the trolls intent on suppressing and attacking the book. One article by Pinyue Lu 鲁品越 entitled "Fang Fang's Diary: An Indefensible Mistake" argues that "Fang Fang profoundly distorts the great anti-epidemic struggle in Wuhan, China."[37] The article places the foreign translation of the diary within the context of China's long history of suffering and humiliation at the hands of Western powers, ultimately emphatically declaring:

> ...no good will come of using Fang Fang's diary against China, since what is being utilized in this case is a political toxin that contains nothing of value.[38]

Although published in English in a peer-reviewed journal published by Taylor & Francis, the article contains broad generalizations (like "Fang Fang has written a book that sets her against the Chinese nation"[39]), full endorsement of viral conspiracy theories claiming that *Wuhan Diary* is a weapon being used to attack China (even though the article was translated and submitted for consideration just four days after the book's initiation publication), and employing slogan-like political rhetoric (such as the concluding call to arms: "Unite the peoples of the world! Oppose the Western politicians who try to split the world through anti-China actions, and build a community of shared future for mankind"[40]).

Even more surprising was the appearance of a series of full-length Chinese-language academic e-books that were published online before the

---

[37] Pinyue Lu (2020) Fang Fang's Diary: An Indefensible Mistake, International Critical Thought, DOI: https://doi.org/10.1080/21598282.2020.1823612

[38] Ibid.

[39] Ibid.

[40] Ibid.

English translation of *Wuhan Diary* was even released on May 15. The first full-length e-book appeared with the English title *Great Wuhan But Bad Diary* (the words "Wuhan" and "Diary" appeared in boldface as if it was an attempt to deceive readers into thinking they were purchasing the actual *Wuhan Diary*). The book was attributed to someone named Fan Ren 凡人, a pseudonym meaning "Average Person," and was uploaded to Amazon UK, US, and Germany, all the regions where *Wuhan Diary* was available for pre-order at that time.[41] Around the same time another full-length e-book entitled *Criticism of Fang Fang's Diary* (*Fang Fang riji pipan* 方方日記批判) written by Feng Chuan 馮川, an assistant researcher at the Wuhan University School of Political Science and Public Administration, began to circulate on WeChat and other platforms. Running at more than a hundred pages, Feng Chuan's book purports to offer "an objective assessment" and "take complete stock" of the book; however, it ultimately ends up being a political hit job under the guise of objective academic scholarship. As the conclusion demonstrates, *Criticism of Fang Fang's Diary* ends up offering a critique no less scathing than the numerous online attacks and articles:

> Although she seems to express a sense of identification with average citizens, Fang Fang's sense of psychological identification with the government and the party-state system is almost non-existent. However, amid our contemporary world of citizen states, to not recognize the central interest of the nation is a betrayal of average citizens and runs the risk of serving the interests of international competitors. In China today under the leadership of the Chinese Communist Party a failure to recognize the government and the party system displays a lack of Chinese political common sense resulting in the individual inevitably falling into the conundrum of binary thinking; from there, one heads in the direction of self-negation and ends up on the road to "spiritual groveling." It begins with the aging of one's structure of knowledge and ends with a tendency that goes against the system, leaving the nation and its people behind. This is not only the most fundamental flaw of *Fang Fang's Diary* but it is also the most damaging aspect of *Fang Fang's Diary*.[42]

---

[41] In August 2020 a new version of Fan Ren's book was released on barnesandnoble.com with a revised cover design that copied the HarperVia cover of *Wuhan Diary*.

[42] Feng Chuan 馮川. *Criticism of Fang Fang's Diary* (*Fang Fang riji pipan* 方方日記批判) e-book, 2020 pgs. 204–105. No publisher listed.

Both books carry on the legacy of political criticism (*zhengzhi pipan* 政治批判), which was so central to the political campaigns of the Mao era, such as the Anti-Rightist Movement and the Cultural Revolution—only now the criticisms are unleashed in a digital cyberspace and immediately disseminated to millions of readers. It is also worth noting that although by this time, the official title of the book had been well established as *Wuhan Diary* in English and *Wuhan riji* 武漢日記 in Chinese, detractors of the book continued to refer to it despairingly as *Fang Fang's Diary*, in keeping with the previously discussed negation of Fang Fang's right to "speak for Wuhan." Both *Great Wuhan But Bad Diary* and *Criticism of Fang Fang's Diary* suddenly appeared online in early May, but one twist I did not expect was that by August they had both been erased from the internet.[43] Amazon no longer listed Fan Ren's e-book for sale and online searches come up with no results, while Feng Chuan's e-book appeared to have been scrubbed from WeChat. In the quickly changing world of the Chinese internet, not only were pro-Fang Fang posts being deleted from the internet, but even evidence of the most malicious pages from the smear campaign against the book seemed to be disappearing. As traces of the digital footprints surrounding the so-called Fang Fang Incident began to fade, the importance of preserving this history became even more pressing.

[43] While Feng Chuan's e-book was deleted from WeChat, it can still be found archived in text form on the website Utopia (Wuyou zhi xiang wangkan 烏有之鄉網刊) under the alternate title *Text, Logic, and Problems with Fang Fang's Diary* (*Fang Fang riji de wenben, luoji-yuwenti* 《方方日記》的文本、邏輯與問題) http://www.wyzxwk.com/Article/yulun/2020/05/417613.html.

CHAPTER 6

Witch Hunt

As the attacks on Fang Fang gained traction, another tactic employed transformed the campaign against the author into a veritable witch hunt aimed at silencing stories and individuals who had publicly defended *Wuhan Diary*. It began with a social media posts by high-profile celebrities and public intellectuals who had come out in defense of the author having their pro-Fang Fang posts being scrubbed from the internet in China. On April 9, just as the troll attacks were raging, controversial television host, film historian, former CCTV talk show host, and public intellectual Cui Yongyuan 崔永元 posted an article entitled "A Lesson for Fang Fang" (Gei Fang Fang shang yi ke 給方方上一課). Over the course of his career, Cui has been at the center of a series of large scandals. Most recently, he was the target of a series of online attacks in 2018 after leaking information about actress Fan Bingbing's 范冰冰[1] film contracts triggered

---

[1] Fan Bingbing is a leading Chinese actress, producer, model, singer, and product spokesperson. During the height of her popularity, Cui Yongyuan leaked photos of her so-called yin-yang contracts 陰陽合約 online. The contracts showed that there were two versions of the same contract, each listed a markedly different salary. The images set off a major scandal that reverberated throughout the Chinese film industry. Fan was detained by Chinese authorities and offered a public apology for tax evasion after her eventual release nearly three months later. She was forced to pay fines in excess of 127 million USD and the government enacted a new taxation scale for high-earning figures in the entertainment industry. The new tax scale resulted in major financial losses for the film industry and made Cui Yongyuan, the whistleblower, the target of widespread online attacks and death threats.

M. Berry, *Translation, Disinformation, and Wuhan Diary*, https://doi.org/10.1007/978-3-031-16859-8_6

a major scandal that rocked the entire Chinese film industry. In "A Lesson for Fang Fang," Cui shared his experience of being targeted and offered suggestions for Fang Fang.

> I deliver this lesson from the perspective of someone who has been through it; someone who has managed to somehow escape with his life from the battlefield of the internet. From my perspective, you are currently only just in the very early phase of this war so be sure not to rashly open fire, preserve your ammunition. Right now you should be looking at the map and listening to suggestions from old combat veterans like us; we have paid a price in blood to learn these lessons.[2]

In his open letter to Fang Fang, the main lessons Cui goes on to outline deal with the futility of responding to the trolls (who just come back in larger numbers with even more attacks) and the futility of suing her detractors for slander (which Fang Fang had been attempting to do). In the wake of being targeted, Cui had attempted both, resulting only in more frustration, delays, and setbacks. Instead, referencing the title of Fang Fang's famously suppressed novel, Cui urges his fellow victim, "From today onward, Fang Fang, forget about your lawsuit, give it a soft burial."[3] In explaining the futility of trying to fight the trolls, Cui also describes the different echelons mobilized for attack. It is a fascinating passage that offers a snapshot of the diverse support these types of cyber campaigns enjoy. As Cui writes:

> They are made up of people from all different backgrounds. Just from those I have encountered, there are professors like Zhang Yiwu from Peking University, Xiao Ying 肖鷹 from Tsinghua University, and Ke Bingsheng 柯柄生 from Agricultural University, there are large numbers of university students from numerous campuses across the country, there is a retired Assistant Commander from the People's Liberation Army who founded his own company while still serving in the military, there is a former pilot from the Chinese Airforce who once knocked a lead aircraft out of the sky while flying as a wingman, judges and public prosecutors in active service, those foul and

---

[2] Cui Yongyuan 崔永元. "A Lesson for Fang Fang" (Gei Fang Fang shang yi ke 給方方上一課). The essay was originally uploaded to Weibo but quickly censored. Fortunately, the article has been reported by numerous other websites and users (often as a jpeg image or even as YouTube style video essay in order to avoid further censorship). The essay can be found here: https://www.xiaxiaoqiang.net/previous-lesson/.html.

[3] Ibid.

utterly corrupt women behind Hong Kong Television, editors-in-chief at major newspapers and magazines, there are traffic police officers, scientists, the children of revolutionaries and officials…and what they all have in common is the fact that they are all utter numbskulls. You could divide them into two categories; one group is just stupid, the other is simply evil.

I won't recall all the battles I fought with them since each and every one ended disastrously.

But now that this elite group has come for you Fang Fang, can you handle them? Are you willing to expend your mental and physical energy and throw away years of your life on them?[4]

"A Lesson for Fang Fang" was also quickly given a "soft burial," scrubbed from the internet and "disappeared." Other voices of support were dealt with in a similar fashion. Award-winning Chinese-American writer Yan Geling 嚴歌苓, a popular figure in the Chinese literary world, published an essay entitled "Hide! Hide! Hide!" 瞞!瞞!瞞! which references Fang Fang (and Fang Fang, in turn, mentions Yan in her diary); the essay decries the tendency in China to cover up and hide, describing how "We have become an amnesiac people. The Nanjing Massacre, the Three Years of Famine, and the Cultural Revolution, we do everything in our power to hide them from ourselves."[5] Of course, like Cui Yongyuan's essay, Yan Geling's "Hide! Hide! Hide!" was also quickly hidden away, targeted by the internet censors and deleted.

Censorship is, of course, a fact of everyday life on the Chinese internet; however, the online suppression of information concerning *Wuhan Diary* was unusual. Some of that suppression should not be viewed as specific to Fang Fang's diary, but to an overall clampdown concerning how information was being policed during the early phase of the COVID-19 outbreak in Wuhan. The control of information surrounding coronavirus can be seen from the very beginning, "on December 30 [2019]…the Health Commission had issued an urgent internal notice that prohibited anyone in the health system from disclosing any information related to the

---

[4] Ibid.

[5] Yan Geling "Hide! Hide! Hide" has been translated by Nicky Harman and is available on the Paper Republic website: https://paper-republic.org/pubs/read/hide-hide-hide/. Fang Fang refers to the essay in the March 16 installment of her diary. (In the English translation of *Wuhan Diary* the Yan Geling essay is translated as "Conceal, conceal, conceal." The Chinese term *man* could also be rendered as muffle.)

coronavirus disease without authorization."[6] Jasper Becker has observed that "Chinese authorities started censoring news of the virus from search engines from 31 December [2019], deleting terms including 'SARS variation', 'Wuhan Seafood Market' and 'Wuhan Unknown Pneumonia'."[7] The later reprimand of the "eight whistleblowers," which included Dr. Li Wenliang and other Wuhan-based physicians like Dr. Ai Fen 艾芬, can all be traced to this clampdown. In *Shutdown: How Covid Shook the World's Economy*, Adam Tooze provided an overview of how the death of Dr. Li Wenliang triggered an immediate public outcry, which was in turn met by swift and even fiercer crackdown:

> Dismay at the regime's mishandling of the pandemic quickly spilled over into more general political demands. On Friday, February 7 [the day of Li Wenliang's death], an open letter by professors of Wuhan's well-regarded university called on the authorities to honor the freedom of expression guaranteed in China's constitution. Another letter addressed to China's National People's Congress by leading intellectuals started by declaring: "We assert, starting today, that no Chinese citizen should be threatened by any state apparatus or political group for his or her speech…The state must immediately cease censoring social media and deleting or blocking accounts." Only weeks earlier, Xi's authority had seemed unquestionable. Now the censors were struggling to prevent web users from posting lyrics from "Do You Hear the People Sing?," *Les Misérables*'s theme tune, which had recently been adopted as an anthem of defiance by protestors in Hong Kong. […] The upsurge of protest was met with tough repression. Censorship went into overdrive. Social media posts were rapidly wiped. Local Wuhan Reporters who dared to post critical video online disappeared.[8]

It was amid this environment of unprecedented censorship and control that transformed what would otherwise be considered a straightforward account of the lockdown into an exposé. As former Weibo employee and China Digital Times editor Eric Liu observed, the model employed to curate online discourse involved not only censorship but also the harnessing of hate campaigns:

[6] Yang, Guobin. *The Wuhan Lockdown*. New York: Columbia University Press: 2021. Pg. 10.

[7] Becker, Jasper. *Made in China: Wuhan, COVID and the Quest for Biotech Supremacy*. London: C. Hurst & Co. 2021. Pg. 265.

[8] Tooze, Adam. *Shutdown: How Covid Shook the World's Economy*. New York: Viking, 2021. Pg. 56.

China invested an unprecedented amount of energy into the control of public discourse during the COVID-19 era and part of this propaganda model necessitated hatred targets. Besides the traditional use of the United States as a target of hatred, they also successfully incited hatred against Chinese who had returned from overseas, which could be described as 'applying poison across a thousand miles.' And then there was hatred towards "traitors to China" and "turncoats," all of which were collectively employed in the attacks against Fang Fang.[9]

It is essential to understand that online attacks against Fang Fang and the entire cat-and-mouse game concerning online posts about *Wuhan Diary* were playing out against a much larger information war being waged in Wuhan, which, in turn, is also situated within the broader historical intersection of censorship and viral outbreaks. We can, for instance, find a unique antecedent in the 2003 SARS outbreak. During that time, information was tightly controlled, dissenting voices were suppressed, and even literary forms that attempted to portray the epidemic, like Hu Fayun's 胡發云 2006 novel *Ruyan@SARS.come* 如焉, were banned. In the case of the 2003 epidemic, Carlos Rojas has even argued that "with SARS these censorship efforts ultimately reinforced the public's association of the disease with the corresponding Sinophone regions. Together these two processes offer a useful model for understanding the relationship between political regimes and processes of community formation and perceptions of national identity."[10] Given the incredible surge in anti-Chinese discrimination globally and rampant politicization of COVID-19, it is interesting to ponder the relationship between these trends and the control of information flow. By all accounts, there was an incredible thrust to shape information about coronavirus during the early phases of the outbreak. According to a BBC report "Novel Coronavirus: The 'Battle to Delete Posts' Beyond Wuhan" published on March 11, 2020,[11] reports, videos, and social media posts on the Wuhan outbreak were already being heavily censored. The independent agency Telegram reported that more than 400

---

[9] Author interview with Eric Liu, May 11, 2021.
[10] Rojas, Carlos. *Homesickness: Culture, Contagion, and National Transformation in Modern China*. Cambridge: Harvard University Press, 2015. Pg. 164.
[11] "Novel Coronavirus: The 'Battle to Delete Posts' Beyond Wuhan" ("Feiyan yiqing: Wuhan zhiwai de 'shantiezhan'") BBC News Chinese Online. March, 11, 2020. https://www.bbc.com/zhongwen/simp/chinese-news-51830859

posts had been deleted during the early phase of the outbreak.[12] And *The New York Times* reported on March 14 that "The Chinese government, eager to claim victory in what China's leader Xi Jinping has described as a 'people's war' against the virus, is leading a sweeping campaign to purge the public sphere of dissent, censoring news reports, harassing citizen journalists and shutting down news sites."[13] Follow-up reporting by *The New York Times* in December of 2020 revealed thousands of internal government directives issued during the early days of the COVID-19; according to the report:

> …censors decided to double down. Warning of the "unprecedented challenge" Dr. Li (Wenliang)'s passing had posed and the "butterfly effect" it may have set off, officials got to work suppressing the inconvenient news and reclaiming the narrative, according to confidential directives sent to local propaganda workers and news outlets.[14]

This thrust to shape and control how the coronavirus narrative was being told had a direct impact on how internet authorities handled Fang Fang's account, which was probably the most widely read non-official source of information about the Wuhan outbreak at the time. According to WeChat Scope, an online portal at the University of Hong Kong which monitors censorship on WeChat, posts and articles including the keyword "Fang Fang" were among the most heavily censored terms during 2020. In the case of Fang Fang, however, not only were articles, posts, and interviews supporting the writer being deleted (not to mention many of Fang Fang's original diary posts), but witch hunt-like tactics were also employed to intimidate and, in some cases, punish her friends and supporters (Fig. 6.1).

As the internet trolls increased their attacks against Fang Fang in early April, several individuals who had posted their support of Fang Fang social media including Professor Liang Yanping 梁艳萍 (Hubei University), poet and Professor Wang Xiaoni 王小妮 (Hainan University), and Liu

---

[12] Ibid.

[13] Hernandez, Javier C. "As China Cracks Down on Coronavirus Coverage, Journalists Fight back" New York Times, March 14, 2020. https://www.nytimes.com/2020/03/14/business/media/coronavirus-china-journalists.html

[14] Raymond Zhong, Paul Mozur, Jeff Kao and Aaron Krolik. "No 'Negative' News: How China Censored the Coronavirus" New York Times, December 19, 2020. https://www.nytimes.com/2020/12/19/technology/china-coronavirus-censorship.html?smid=em-share

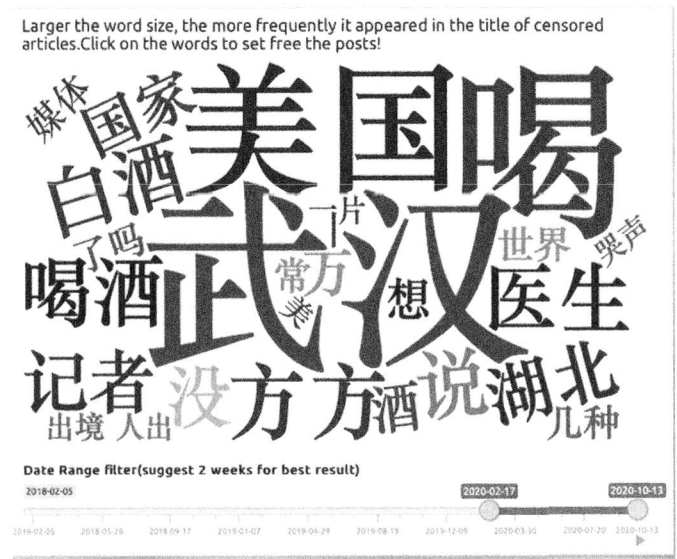

Fig. 6.1 This WordClouds image was created using the platform WeChat Scope, which provides visualizations of frequently censored terms on WeChat. This image, tracing the most censored terms from 2/17/20 through 10/13/20, shows Fang Fang prominently displayed in the center bottom

Chuan-e 劉川鄂 (Hubei University) all became targets. In the case of Professors Liang Yanping and Wang Xiaoni, online attackers began to demand their respective universities launch official investigations into their online speech. In the case of Wang Xiaoni, the online pressure was so great that the official Weibo account of Hainan University posted a public notice on April 30, 2020, that read: "Statement: In response to internet users who have raised concerns over the issue of improper speech published by Wang Xiaoni, who is a retired professor from our university, the school has already established a special working group to investigate these charges." The statement made it clear that the investigation was being fueled by allegations made by netizens.

When Hubei University did not immediately take action against Liang Yanping, the trolls began to threaten university administrators, saying that they too would be targeted if action was not taken. Then on April 26, 2020, Hubei University announced it was launching a formal investigation into Professor Liang's social media posts. Ultra-leftist Weibo users and ultra-nationalist websites like Red China celebrated the decision with comments like "after the tireless efforts of countless patriotic netizens, Hubei University has, after a long period of hesitation, finally announced [an investigation into Liang Yanping]…some say that the phenomena surrounding Fang Fang's so-called "diary" and the various incidents that have spun out from the controversy have torn Chinese society apart. This is utter nonsense. Yu Nie 余涅 wholeheartedly believes that thanks to the broad masses of the people who, inspired by their fervent patriotic passion, have risen up to monitor the actions of members of that 'fortunate generation' who have abused their power, political identification amongst members of Chinese society will become even more stable, China will become a more unified country, and China's future will be even more glorious!"[15] Part of the internet trolls' tactics was not simply to attack Fang Fang's supporters through social media posts, but also to use their power to voice complaints, file grievances, and demand various investigations be launched. In the case of Liang Yanping, it was not only her pro-Fang Fang posts which came under scrutiny; detractors also combed through her entire social media history, digging through years of old posts on Weibo; they found "objectionable" posts concerning her stance on the Hong Kong anti-extradition movement and the Nanjing Massacre. It would actually be those older posts which would eventually result in Professor Liang Yanping being removed from teaching and stripped from her membership to the Chinese Communist Party. The trolls, seemingly, had won.[16]

But the witch hunt continued; Wang Xiaoni, one of the leading poets of her generation and a professor emeritus from Hainan University, was also subjected to repeated attacks and calls for an official investigation. Founder of the Goethe-Institut China, sinologist Michael Kahn-Ackermann, who served as the German translator of *Wuhan Diary*, also came under attack, as of course did I. Along the way, more and more trolls began using the word *gongzhi* 公知 (abbreviated form of 公共知識分子), "public intellectual,"

---

[15] "Some Remarks on the Investigation into Hubei University Professor Liang Yanping" ("Tantan Hubei daxue diaocha Liang Yanping jiaoshou" 〈談談湖北大學調查梁艷萍教授〉) on Red China (RedChinaCn.net) on April 28, 2020. (No author is formally listed, but based on the text, the author seems to be Yu Nie 余涅.) http://redchinacn.org/forum.php?mod=viewthread&tid=16793&extra=page%3D1

[16] Professor Liang Yanping's investigation was widely covered in both the Chinese and Western media. For more on the investigation, see https://www.scmp.com/news/china/politics/article/3089929/chinese-professor-banned-teaching-over-hong-kong-protest.

6 WITCH HUNT   95

as a derogatory term to attack more liberal-minded Chinese intellectuals like Wang Xiaoni and Liang Yanping. In January 2021, Sima Nan, Yam Bear Six, and other critics of Fang Fang launched a series of attacks against Jia Qianqian 賈淺淺, who had been credited a co-author of book with Fang Fang in 2019.[17] The attacks against Jia were not only directed at her connection to Fang Fang, but also targeted her "inferior literary talent" and accused her and her father, veteran writer Jia Pingwa 賈平凹, of nepotistic practices. For years, savvy Chinese netizens had engaged in a game of linguistic inversion, using terms like *bei hexie* 被和諧 (been harmonized) to critique the government's call for voices that have been silenced under the call for the establishment of a "harmonious society" (*hexie shehui* 和諧社會), but now it was the ultra-leftists offering a revisionist interpretation of the language. Once respected and looked up to in society, the very term public intellectual was now inverted as a politically incorrect label (*gongzhi*) to attack individuals who dared to speak out.

To show just how deep the rabbit hole goes, consider the following: one of my senior colleagues at UCLA decided to devote one session of her Spring 2020 seminar on COVID-19 to *Wuhan Diary*. This colleague, a US citizen and full professor at UCLA, happened to concurrently hold an honorary professorship at a top research university in China; when a faculty member from that Chinese university heard that she was teaching *Wuhan Diary* (at UCLA!), he "reported" my colleague to the campus authorities in China, triggering an investigation! My colleague decided to resign from her post in China. And then there was a prominent Chinese public intellectual who during the early phase of the outbreak had published extensively and enthusiastically in support of Fang Fang and her diary. When I reached out to him/her about the possibility of contributing a blurb for the English version of *Wuhan Diary*, his/her response sent chills down my spine: "I should write something and I really want to write something…but right now there is nothing I dare say or do. I hope you can forgive me…" The ellipsis trailing at the end of his/her text spoke of such pain. The witch hunt was effectively silencing Fang Fang's supporters. I caught another glimpse of this form of self-censorship when a group of Chinese undergraduate

---

[17] Even the fact that Jia Qianqian "co-authored" a book with Fang Fang is a rather tenuous claim meant to overexaggerate the relationship between Jia and Fang. In reality, the book in question was a collection of essays entitled *Our Fathers* (*Women de fuqin* 我們的父親) published by Wuhan University Press, which featured contributions from 25 contributors; Fang Fang and Jia Qianqian (along with Cui Yongyuan) happen to be the three contributors highlighted on the book's cover.

students who were part of a theater troupe approached me about the possibility of adapting *Wuhan Diary* into a radio play; they wanted me to help them get in touch with Fang Fang; however, just a few days later they wrote back to me: because of the political controversy that had erupted, they decided to cancel their radio play; the diary had become too "sensitive" to take on. Another group of UCLA students contacted me about translating a collection of testimonies about the Wuhan lockdown into English; they too abandoned their plan after they witnessed the online vitriol Fang Fang was facing. All of these examples further illustrate the validity of Guobin Yang's earlier observation about how attacking Fang Fang had a much more pervasive and chilling impact on silencing other witnesses, activists, and other forms of commemoration.

Of course, the most tenacious and brutal witch hunt was reserved for Fang Fang herself. Her numerous publications and social media history were subjected to unprecedented scrutiny; details about her history of international travel, real estate holdings, and private life were made public; her home address was leaked online; her adult daughter's name and information was posted on the internet; numerous official complaints were filed about her; and, of course, the death threats and personal attacks online persisted. Many of the attacks were reminiscent of the type of political persecution that was ubiquitous in Chinese society during the Cultural Revolution. Born in 1955, Fang Fang had spent her formative years growing up during the Cultural Revolution and she clearly saw the similarities. Throughout the persecution campaign, Fang Fang has consistently referred to her detractors as "ultra-leftists" (*jizuo* 極左), a label leftover from the "ten years of internal chaos" used to refer to ultra-nationalists who employ Maoist rhetoric and tactics reminiscent of the Cultural Revolution. Once can clearly see the legacy of the Cultural Revolution in the social media posts, the political views emphasized in their essays and publications, and the very tactics they employ. The "witch hunt," which was launched to persecute Fang Fang's supporters, is a case in point. During the Cultural Revolution, "guilt by association" and attacking individuals merely for their contacts and family background were common affairs. In the case of Fang Fang, these tactics were not only employed, but celebrated.

Eventually, the Cultural Revolution seemed to come full circle. Anti-Fang Fang political posters produced in the style of socialist realist propaganda posters began to appear on Weibo and flood the Chinese internet. Highly reminiscent of the denunciation posters used to criticize the Gang of Four, these dehumanizing images portrayed Fang Fang as the "enemy of the people," deserving of society's scorn and attacks. One such image labeled "Down with the imperialist running dog and traitor to China, Fang Fang" featured an overweight Fang Fang with exaggerated features, including a dog's tail (an example of zoomorphism no doubt intended to accentuate her identity as a true "running dog" in service of the Western imperialist powers) as she cowers on the ground writing her diary; meanwhile a trio of fit, young "Little Pink" heroes tower over her in a threatening stance. A sea of glorious red flags flutter against the three Little Pink heroes while an ominous sea of black with jagged teeth-like edges surrounds Fang Fang. Unlike during the Cultural Revolution when the holy revolutionary trinity was inevitably made up of model representatives from the three classes of worker, peasant, and soldier, they are here represented by a new incarnation of Chinese heroes. Wielding a calligraphy brush, a ballpoint pen, and a red lantern (another Cultural Revolution reference to the famous model opera *The Red Lantern*), these are revolutionary heroes for the new age of "socialism with Chinese characteristics." And, in case there had been any doubt, posts also began appearing on WeChat, making it clear that the intimidation and persecution of Fang Fang's supporters was a clear-cut strategy being actively employed. One such post a friend sent me on April 29, 2020, included the cryptic message:

> *Who will be the next one?*
> *Keep watching Fang Fang's circle of friends and you will see!*
> *Little Red Soldiers April 29, 2020.*

The "next one" of course referred to the next target of their online campaign after Liang Yanping, Wang Xiaoni, and others. The campaign against Fang Fang had evolved into a true cyber witch hunt aimed at hunting down and weeding out those prominent public figures who had stood up for Fang Fang and *Wuhan Diary*. The campaign had evolved in other ways as well: what had begun as a cyber-attack started to spill into the real world. Besides the very real consequences faced by people like Professor Liang Yanping, the threat of real physical violence to Fang Fang seemed to creep closer. Thugs threw bricks over the wall into the compound where she lived and yet another ghost from the Cultural Revolution returned: the big character poster.

In mid-April these denunciation posters began to appear posted in public spaces near Fang Fang's home. The posters harkened back to the political speak of the Mao era and threatened Fang Fang with violence. One anonymous handwritten big character poster from April 15, 2020, stated:

> *An Open Letter to Fang Fang*
>
> *Fang Fang, she who consumes steamed buns soaked in human blood, was born into a New China, raised under the Red Flag and has enjoyed all of the various benefits and treatment of the state system, has now done terrible things which have deeply harmed our nation with false claims. No need for Fang Fang to ask who I am, I know who I am, I am a peasant from the countryside who "yesterday was still in the fields planting peanuts." Though that may be the case, this has not stopped me from coming to Wuhan; I have made my way here to carry out a crusade against you Fang Fang to express my hatred and anger for what you have done.*
>
> *I hereby forcefully request that Fang Fang turn every bit of her property and assets to the state; then she should either shave her head and take up the vows of a Buddhist nun or kill herself in order to repent for her sins and crimes against the people of this nation. If this is not done I will take it upon myself as an individual to carry out justice in accordance with the Chinese people's ancient and pure method of chivalrous justice (xiayi); the attack against Fang Fang be both verbal and physical.*

The reference to Fang Fang consuming "steamed buns soaked in human blood" 人血饅頭 is an allusion to Lu Xun, the father of modern Chinese literature and author of "A Madman's Diary," which I earlier juxtaposed against *Wuhan Diary*. The image of "steamed buns soaked in human blood" is from Lu Xun's iconic short story "Medicine" ("Yao" 藥), in which a young boy suffering from tuberculosis is urged by his family to gobble down a blood-soaked bun, which is touted as a miracle cure. The blood comes from the body of a recently executed revolutionary who died trying to "save" China. In the end, the boy dies; his family's superstitious belief in a miracle cure proves just as ineffective as the revolutionary's efforts to reform China. The metaphor of the blood-soaked bun is not accidental; during the height of the attacks against Fang Fang, it was one of the most frequently employed cultural references. Fang Fang (and even I) was repeatedly characterized as consuming steamed buns soaked in the blood of the victims of Wuhan. In the case of Fang Fang, however, the employment of the Lu Xun steamed bun reference is a corruption. Whereas Fang Fang attempted to "wake people up" with her diary (or destroy the iron house, if we use Lu Xun's imagery), her detractors have inverted the logic, transforming *her* into the oppressor, the system, the cannibal feasting on the bodies of her compatriots.

However, it is precisely owing to these sloppy metaphors, broad generalizations, and black-and-white simplifications which have allowed Fang
Fang's detractors to so successfully turn the tide of public opinion against
her. Another online detractor posted:

> As the Fang Fang Diary Incident has developed, we are now at the point
> where it has led to our nation and even overseas Chinese to face embarrass-
> ment, difficulties, and even threats against their lives. The people of our
> nation have only now just recovered from the sadness and pain of the Grave
> Sweeping Festival and now the last thing we need is to face the tremendous
> hurt caused by the international distribution of Fang Fang's Diary. Since it
> is like a rat trap, our government is clearly facing the hurt of betrayal yet
> there is nothing they can do to Fang Fang. But we as citizens should at this
> moment rise up and, just like during the Battle of Huaihai, when tens of
> thousands of everyday citizens brought their carts to help with the war
> effort, we too should form a tide of public opinion to speak a resounding
> "NO!" to the actions of betrayal and hurt that Fang Fang has caused our
> nation. We should launch a punitive campaign to forcefully expose and criti-
> cize her. As a peasant I have now temporarily put aside my work in the fields
> and my family responsibilities to rush to Wuhan in order to take care of
> these state affairs.

Tuo Wang has characterized the big character posters of the Cultural
Revolution period as following a set formula, which usually consisted of
"quotations of Mao, the name of the person being discussed in the poster,
tangential evidence of him or her being a counter-revolutionary, a call for
action against the person, and more praises of Mao."[18] In this contemporary update of the big character poster, Mao has of course dropped out,
replaced by references to "New China," "the Red Flag," and the "Chinese
people," which now serve as the ideological arbiters of truth and author-
ity; but the other components of the letter—singling out Fang Fang by
name, listing the evidence of her "crimes," and calling for punishment—
are all there. Additionally, like the Cultural Revolution-era posters, in
which "the writer did not sign his or her real name at the end,"[19] these
anti-Fang Fang posters were also anonymous. But most striking were the
calls for violence, which are here justified by both lofty ideas of nationalism

---

[18] Tuo Wang. *The Cultural Revolution and Overacting: Dynamics Between Politics and Performance.* Lanham: Lexington Books, 2014. Pg. 34.
[19] Ibid. Pg. 34.

and more traditional conceptions of "exacting justice" as understood through folk tales and martial arts novels.

As big character posters reappeared, Cultural Revolution-style anti-Fang Fang propaganda posters spread on WeChat, misogynistic threats and attacks against Fang Fang proliferated online, and her close friends, collaborators, and supporters became targeted in an ever-widening witch hunt, many China watchers were struck with an ominous feeling. A Hong Kong vlogger posted a video on YouTube entitled "Reading the Top Ten Characteristics of the Cultural Revolution 2.0: The Struggle Session Against Fang Fang's *Wuhan Diary* and Hong Kong's Future."[20] One by one, journalists, bloggers, and Chinese public intellectuals began alternately referring to the campaign against *Wuhan Diary* as the Cultural Revolution 2.0, the Cultural Revolution Redux, the New Cultural Revolution, or China's Digital Cultural Revolution.[21] However, the truly strange part of this remixed version of the Cultural Revolution was the utter and complete absence of any true "revolution." Decades after Mao's revolutionary project, the China of 2020 is now the land of "socialism with Chinese characteristics," perhaps better phrased as "capitalism with authoritarian characteristics"; it is the land of AI surveillance, mega corporations like Alibaba, skyscrapers, and smartphones; and yet, here amid a pandemic a strange, post-revolutionary fervor is unleashed. "The people" are given a new class enemy: a counter-revolutionary, entitled intellectual colluding with the "American imperialists" to sabotage, what exactly? The socialist project? The battle against the coronavirus? The Chinese dream? Truth itself? Perhaps the darkest and most terrifying part of the so-called leftists' attacks are their vacuity: an opportunistic appropriation of a bygone revolutionary fervor in the service of "the good story." Like the suppression of books deemed politically incorrect during the Cultural Revolution, the ultimate target of this witch hunt was the book itself. After Fang Fang had originally signed contracts with publishers in China and Hong Kong, official publication of the Chinese edition of *Wuhan Diary* was abruptly halted. Publishers in China refused to reprint older works or publish new works by Fang Fang, effectively banning her from

---

[20] https://www.youtube.com/watch?v=8tlEKYQ2asE
[21] https://thediplomat.com/2020/04/chinas-digital-cultural-revolution/

the Chinese market.[22] And in another sign that the effort to suppress the book was extending beyond China's own borders, even some of the international publishers of *Wuhan Diary* reported receiving pressure from various agencies in China to halt publication. Writing in 2022, more than two years after she completed her online blog about the pandemic, Fang Fang wrote about the lingering impact the campaign targeting her was still having on her life and career:

> I am unable to print or publish any of my writings within China, I am pro-hibited from participating in any literary or public events, my name is not allowed to appear in any mainstream publications, professional literary crit-ics have been completely banned from carrying out research on my work, and even when independent or self-published media entities publish my essays they are either shut down or blocked. I repeatedly receive phone calls from higher-ups reminded me not to accept any foreign interview requests, that all my communications are being monitored and controlled. Whenever I go out, I receive phone calls 'checking up' on me to ask where I am. Not only that, the ultra-leftists attacking me have even used the slogan 'besiege the enemy stronghold in order to attack the reinforcements,' to describe their campaign of exposing the names of all people (and their family mem-bers) who support me online and attacking them. If those individuals or their relatives are found to have ever made any purportedly 'inappropriate statements' or had a history of any speech or actions that violated certain regulations, the government takes swift punitive measures against them. These types of underhanded 'guilt-by-association' tactics have left me and my friends in an extremely precarious situation. Once these vicious forces coming from outside the government reach a consensus with those in power and join forces, what else can I possibly say.[23]

Of course, one of the core facets of the Cultural Revolution between 1966 and 1976 was the way in which the movement harnessed culture itself as a political and ideological weapon. Problematic cultural works,

---

[22] In an interview with Asahi Shimbun, Fang Fang told a reporter that she is unable to publish her latest novel and other books in China, which she described as a form of "cold violence." Fang Fang stated: "Publishing houses across the nation suddenly stopped issuing my books…It is natural that authorities have exerted pressure on them by some means." Kanako Miyajima. "Author of 'Wuhan Diary' now finds herself muzzled in China" The Asahi Shimbun, December 15, 2020. http://www.asahi.com/ajw/articles/13988776.

[23] Fang Fang. "I Will Face it All with No Misgivings: After *Wuhan Diary*" in *Wuhan Diary: Dispatches from a Quarantined City*. Revised Paperback edition. HarperVia, 2022. pg. 364–365.

beginning with *Hai Rui Dismissed from Office*, were suppressed and attacked; meanwhile a new crop of revolutionary works "correct in orientation" (or, using the political lingo of 2020, we could describe them as works imbued with "positive energy") came to dominate—revolutionary model operas, revolutionary ballets, propaganda posters, and revolutionary anthems praising Mao. Naturally, much has changed since the revolutionary fervor of the 1960s: the revolutionary categories of "workers, peasants, and soldiers" have been replaced by Little Pinks, wolf warriors, and the 50 Cent Army (*wumaodang* 五毛黨); cold war-era networks for disseminating propaganda (newspapers, radio, film, political directives sent down through work units, etc.) have been updated with new online tools (political apps like Xuexi 學習, social media platforms like Weibo and WeChat, streaming sites like Youku and Bilibili, and a social credit system that rewards "proper" behavior); and big character posters and in-person struggle sessions have been tossed aside for "human-flesh search engines" and online hate campaigns. Of course, thanks to more than four decades of opening up and reform, Chinese society today is a much more diverse, dynamic, and international society than five decades ago. But it is precisely the hindsight of such progress that makes the revisionist slip back towards Cultural Revolution-era discourse all the more uncanny. Who could have imagined that half a century later, as the witch hunt against Fang Fang raged and a new cyber Cultural Revolution quickly took shape, *Wuhan Diary*, an everyday chronicle written during the early days of a global pandemic, would somehow inconceivably slip into the world of pop culture? Once again, culture itself would be weaponized.

CHAPTER 7

Pop Goes Fang Fang?

On April 15 a PhD student at Harvard University sent me a link to a rap song about Fang Fang that had appeared on the internet. A rap song about Fang Fang? After all the attacks, rumors, and trolling, I had come to expect the unexpected, but a rap song? The whole thing felt surreal. While I was initially surprised by the appearance of a Fang Fang diss song, I shouldn't have been. In a world where everything, sooner or later, becomes a meme, it was perhaps inevitable that Fang Fang too would enter the realm of popular culture. The sudden emergence of Fang Fang in pop culture also speaks to the ways in which, in the online world, pop culture has become a ubiquitous and essential component of political theater. What would the 2020 US election have looked like without the inundation of memes, *Saturday Night Live* parody sketches, GIFs, deep-fake video parodies like *Sassy Justice*, and political cartoons? For Chinese netizens who have grown weary of simple top-down official propaganda, messaging emerging from the portal of pop culture can, ironically enough, add a layer of what is perceived to be "truth legitimacy" to critical discourse, as it presents the messages in a context that feels organic and seemingly originates from an outpouring of grassroots public sentiment. This can be heightened by harnessing popular genres like rap, which have a history of speaking truth to power, criticizing social injustice, and representing a discourse that runs counter to official state media. Guobin Yang has also discussed the key role that "playful political engagement" and

© The Author(s), under exclusive license to Springer Nature
Switzerland AG 2022
M. Berry, *Translation, Disinformation, and Wuhan Diary*,
https://doi.org/10.1007/978-3-031-16859-8_7

"cultural skills" have in cyber-nationalism.[1] He has observed how the new generation of "Little Pink" nationalists are millennials; they "are China's digital natives, immersed as they are in a digital culture of online gaming and fandom communities and on social media."[2] With many of the attacks on *Wuhan Diary* being driven by this younger generation of cyber warriors, as the controversy against the book mounted, the turn to popular culture must have been inevitable. By adopting this culture of play, these pop culture attacks also made the political messages aimed at Fang Fang more palpable and accessible to less politically engaged netizens. By reducing Fang Fang to a meme, everyone could now be a part of the attacks against her.

The song that the student from Harvard sent me, my first taste of Fang Fang's appearance in pop music, was entitled "Round on the Inside, Square on the Outside" (Neiyuan waifang 内圆外方), with "square" (*fang* 方) referring to Fang Fang's name. The music and lyrics were attributed to a composer using the pen name Bo Peep and the lyrics read like a summary of the political campaign against Fang Fang:

> There is a woman named Fang Fang in Hubei
> But Fang Fang seems a little flustered recently
> She seems to have become enamored with the fragrance of so-called freedom and democracy
> Why are people raising their rifles against her cries to "speak out from a sense of justice"
> What kind of decent person keeps a diary on the internet
> Proofreading and translation of a book in just over ten days
> [Photos] of abandoned cellphones all over the ground all came from a friend's' text
> Claiming you live a modest life like the common people while living a $20 million dollar villa
> …
> "The world is enveloped in darkness and Fang Fang is the only light"
> Those who oppose her are all "Ultra-Leftists" or must have a brain injury
> They dare not speak the truth because there are guns up against them
> How could Wuhan allow you to sully the city with your dirt?

---

[1] See Guobin Yang's chapter on "Performing Cyber-Nationalism in Twenty-First Century China: The Case of Diba Expedition" in Liu, Hailong ed. *From Cyber-Nationalism to Fandom Nationalism: The Case of Diba Expedition in China*. New York: Routledge, 2020. Pgs. 1–12, especially the section on "Cultural skills and cyber-nationalism" pgs. 6–7.

[2] Ibid. Pg. 7.

...

This bigoted performance was selected in a way to suit her audience
Using her old ways to fan the flames of public opinion
No matter it be real of fake, you won't have any doubts once you check out the
comments section [of her posts]
She doesn't need to take responsibility because it's just a diary
...
And with every drop of ink you cause another national scar
I'm sure they'll give you an award for writing a new generation of Scar
Literature
As you insist on pretending to be the face of those who speak the truth!
But once all the rot fades it will be revealed that you have been swimming naked
all along
...
If you want to play tricks on us you better try harder
You don't even deserve to be counted among "the persecuted"
...
People thought you were like Wu Song, but now you turn out to be a shareholder
in our national betrayal
...
That's right, the curtain has already fallen on your era
The new generation of young people will be the ones to carry the awesome burden
of strengthening our nation
...

The lyric video for the song was uploaded to Weibo on April 12, 2020; uploaded to YouTube with shoddy machine-generated English subtitles on April 13, 2020; and quickly went viral on Chinese streaming sites.[3] The lyrics effectively include references to all the major allegations against Fang Fang's book that had been targeted both by trolls and in more mainstream Chinese media outlets. These include attack lines aimed at (1) the legitimacy of the book as a "diary"; (2) the scandal over the fast turnaround in terms of translation, proofreading, and production; (3) the controversy regarding a photo of abandoned cellphones; (4) a reference to investigative reports into Fang Fang's finances and "luxury housing"; (5)

---

[3] Although the video is dated April 2, 2020, lines like "Proofreading and translation of a book in just over ten days" clearly indicate that it could not have been produced on that date because news of the book's international release did not appear online until approximately one week later. It was more likely produced on or just before 4/12/2020, which is when the video was uploaded to YouTube.

allegations that she is pandering to her audience; (6) claiming that she has a "persecution complex"; and (7) claims that her diary will hurt both the Chinese nation and overseas Chinese all over the world. As Chang Liu observed in her discussion of the diss song: "The opposition to Fang Fang's diary reveals the nationalist youth's distrust of those who do not share their views, especially the Chinese intellectual elite. In their eyes, morality is contingent on loyalty to the nation and country."[4] It is curious that a professionally produced song was written, performed, and uploaded to numerous social media platforms within days of the controversy surrounding the international publication of *Wuhan Diary* hit the internet. (Ironic considering the multiple allegations that "lightspeed" productions imply political conspiracy.) There is also a strange disconnect between the smooth R&B stylings of the music and the vocal track, which highlights a deep, sultry, female voice singing in a style just between rap and spoken word, and the content of the lyrics, which is essentially a crass political hit job. While on the surface this mismatch between content and form appears out of place, I would argue that it is precisely this absurd pairing that, in itself, attempts to strengthen a kind of messaging which pairs Fang Fang's diary with the absurd and ridiculous. In other words, it isn't just the content of the lyrics that are attacking the author, but the form itself effectively drags a serious literary attempt to engage with a terrible viral outbreak into the realm of sensationalist tabloids and bubble-gum pop.

Just a few weeks later on April 28, 2020, a second anti-Fang Fang pop song was simultaneously uploaded to various online streaming platforms like YouTube and Bilibili. This song was entitled "Literary Scum: Diss Fang Fang," using the term "literary scum" (*wenzha* 文渣), as a pun for the more common curse word *renzha* (人渣), "human scum" or "dregs of society." The lyrics are quite similar to the previous song, with lines like:

> *You call me an ultra-leftist*
> *All you do is condemn us in speech and writing*
> *While our tax money pay your rent, you ungrateful bitch*
> *Are you kidding me?*
> *You're a high official who is now an empty nester*
> *Your kids have immigrated abroad*

---

[4] Chang Liu. "Chinese Young Nationalists amid The COVID-19 Pandemic: A Rap against A "Diary" online essay published on the New School Transregional Center for Democratic Studies," July 20, 2020. https://blogs.newschool.edu/tcds/2020/07/20/chinese-young-nationalists-amid-the-covid-19-pandemic-a-rap-against-a-diary/

And don't even bother wiping the blood you sucked away from your mouth
But you still fucking take it
On the brink of exploding
This despicable worm starts to wiggle around again
And you call yourself a writer!
As if thinking cures cowardice
Your contemptable fate has been destroyed by our courage
Look at that diary witch
Sitting on her high horse as a "Chairperson"
Still sharpening the knife to carry out her assassinations

Like "Round on the Inside, Square on the Outside" which was only credited to an unknown writer/composer working under the pseudonym Bo Peep, there are no singers or songwriters credited for "Literary Scum"; like the vast majority of the online attacks, these "diss songs" were also anonymous.[5] Though these songs came from anonymous sources and the videos were essentially lyric videos with only generic graphics and no images of the performers, they still had a considerable impact. "Round on the Inside, Square on the Outside" racked up more than two million views on Bilibili within just a few months of release and by December of 2020 had over ten million views. And these were only two of the more popular of the many "diss videos" uploaded to attack Fang Fang; others included a viral video of Jay Z and Alicia Keys singing "Empire State of Mind" in concert with vocal track re-dubbed in Chinese with anti-Fang Fang lyrics.

Collectively what this series of anti-Fang Fang rap songs brings to light is not only the tension between content and form, but also the uncanny juxtaposition between the rap genre, which is usually known for its iconoclastic, anti-establishment stance (i.e., "Fight the Power"), and the lyrics used here, which are instead a political throwback to the Cultural Revolution which reinforces existing power structures, injected with contemporary slang. What really comes through in these songs and the strange tension imbedded within is a game of political inversion. While serving as Chair of the Hubei Writers Association Fang Fang was certainly regarded by many as a "state writer." However, with the publication of *Soft Burial*

---

[5] Bo Peep released a second political diss song in December 2020 targeting Australian prime minister Scott Morrison as a response to the deteriorating state of Sino-Austrian relations. For more on Bo Peep's follow-up single, see Bryan Grogan's article "Chinese Rapper's Diss Track Aims at Austrian Prime Minister Scott Morrison" in RADII, December 6, 2020. https://radiichina.com/bo-peep-scott-morrison/.

and later *Wuhan Diary*, she came to be regarded by some as a writer who was not upholding the status quo, but challenging it. Now regarded as the usurper, Fang Fang was targeted with rap songs, which positioned her as a privileged and out-of-touch cadre exploiting the pain of the masses for her own benefit. On the surface, the rap songs seemed to function as they should, as a series of grassroots voices intent on challenging inequalities and exposing social ills. The only problem is that the roles have been inverted: Fang Fang is no longer a government cadre; she is writing as an individual and it is *her* diary that is exposing social ills, challenging political norms, and calling for change; at the same time, the rap form, while still pretending to be a voice of "dissent,"⁶ is now essentially commandeered to serve the interests of deeply ingrained political structures. This shift is not unique to the case of Fang Fang, but is a widely observed trend in Chinese rap. As Yi-Ling Liu, writing for the BBC, has observed: "in stark contrast to the longstanding tradition of counter-culturalism and racial protest that has defined American hip-hop, the politics these rappers are asserting has a distinctly, one-noted nationalist tone."⁷

In addition to the pop songs and music videos attacking the writer, anti-Fang Fang skits, clips, poems, and other videos were rampant on the Chinese internet starting in April 2020. One post from August 9, 2020, by Weibo user "ZBV" featured a video clip with the hashtag "#COVID-19 cases in the USA have exceeded 5 million" and a short post:

> The author of *American Diary* hears from a friend:
> In the area around Washington,
> There are abandoned guns everywhere,
> Spread out all over the ground.⁸

The satirical post uses reimagined details from Fang Fang's account, in this case yet another reference to the picture of abandoned cellphones, to criticize rising COVID-19 cases, gun violence, and social unrest in the

---

⁶ Some of the songs even go so far as to "censor" sensitive words in the lyrics by employing homonyms or asterisks in place of potentially controversial content, a move that I would argue is a performative intervention to make the songs "appear more subversive."

⁷ Yi-Ling Liu. "Why Chinese rappers don't fight the power" BBC. November 6, 2019. https://www.bbc.com/culture/article/20191106-why-chinese-rappers-dont-fight-the-power

⁸ The original Chinese text reads: 《美国日记》作者听朋友说: 华盛顿一带m, 无主枪支, 满地都是.

United States. The attached video featured a clip from the blockbuster Stephen Chow 周星馳 comedy *The Mermaid* (*Meirenyu* 美人鱼), but the dialogue was redubbed to mock America's high number of COVID-19 cases and the lack of government response.[9] It is in posts like this that allegations of Fang Fang's *Wuhan Diary* being "weaponized" by the United States against China are not only fully endorsed but now employed to attack America's shortcomings in handling the pandemic. What we see is, in fact, yet another inversion. *Wuhan Diary* is now not only falsely accused of being weaponized by America to hurt China, but it is being actively weaponized by Chinese trolls to attack the United States.

Fang Fang attacks even made it into the world of digital online art; one disturbing image entitled Crown a Jester (*Wei nongchen jiamian* 為弄臣加冕) was uploaded to Weibo as part of a set of seven images (other images featured satirical takes on Donald Trump, the death of George Floyd, America's response to COVID-19, and the Hong Kong National Security law). The images were uploaded by Wuheqilin (烏合麒麟), a graduate of Art Institute of Changchun University who has become popular online for his CG works of political satire, which even earned him the moniker "Wolf Warrior Artist" (zhanlang huashi 戰狼畫師). In Crown a Jester, Wuheqilin portrays Fang Fang as a kneeling court jester with sloppily smeared face paint, offering a blood-soaked book labeled "Lie Diary" to an American general sitting on a throne. The general prepares to reward Fang Fang's loyalty with a spiked crown tied to a chain (which is more reminiscent of a dog collar), no doubt a symbol that her servitude to the American military and political powers is now absolute and complete. In the background are an army of international reporters armed with cameras and microphones who are enraptured by the spectacle. In what is an uncanny twist to Lu Xun's iconic description of an execution witnessed by a crowd of numb spectators, here the implied act of murder is of China itself as Fang Fang willingly hands over the butcher's knife to America as the international media circles around to celebrate the spectacle. It is, no doubt, a powerful and disturbing image; but it is also an image that uncritically endorses typical anti-Fang Fang talking points. Implicit within the image is the internalization of months of attacks on *Wuhan Diary*, the notion that her diary is filled with lies, the allegation that she was working in

---

[9] Other popular parody videos of *Wuhan Diary* employed clips and screenshots from Jiang Wen's 姜文 film *The Hidden Man* (*Xiebuyazheng* 邪不壓正) to mock Fang Fang with lines like "What kind of person writes a diary online!?".

complicity with the US government, the charge that she was willingly handing America a sharp knife to hurt China, and the belief that everything she has done has been to win international fame, profit, and glory. In that sense, whereas "Round on the Inside, Square on the Outside" and "Literary Scum" were able to condense the anti-Fang Fang talking points into the four-minute pop song format, Crown a Jester was able to distill the major elements of the controversy into a single image.

Crown a Jester even won the praise of none other than Zhang Yiwu of Peking University, who reposted a short video profile of the artist by the *Global Times* on Weibo with the comment:

> A young artist has produced some really fascinating images; it is rare to see someone use his own unique style to satirize those forces working against China and the Chinese people. The style of his images is quite powerful, especially his work Crown a Jester, which is a forward-thinking work. This young man's powers of expression are really quite something.[10]

In his own interview with the *Global Times*, the artist Wuheqilin positions his artwork as an act of resistance. He states that "as external forces invade our sphere of public opinion and invade our culture, more people need to stand up and speak out, using methods like this to resist what is happening." Wuheqilin also directly connected the rise in political art like his own to the coronavirus outbreak stating, "more people have realized from the COVID-19 epidemic that patriotism is not something shameful. The country is worth loving and needs every one of us to safeguard it."[11] But like the diss songs and rap parodies discussed earlier, in Crown a Jester one can also observe the way in which anti-Fang Fang discourse has self-positioned itself as a voice of resistance (Fig. 7.1).

But perhaps one of the most shocking and unexpected turns in the pop culture persecution of Fang Fang was an incident that occurred on April 16. Wei Lei 魏雷, a prominent Tai Chi master based in Chengdu usually referred to as Lei Lei 雷雷, stepped into the ring with Fang Fang. Founder of the school of "Thunder God Tai Chi 雷公太極," Lei Lei posted a short 1-minute and 39-second video where he offered a public denunciation of

[10] From a June 21, 2020, post to Zhang Yiwu's Weibo account.
[11] Li Lei. "'Wolf Warrior' artist strives to use new art to spread truth and inspire patriotism" in The Global Times; June 18, 2020. https://www.globaltimes.cn/page/202006/1192217.shtml

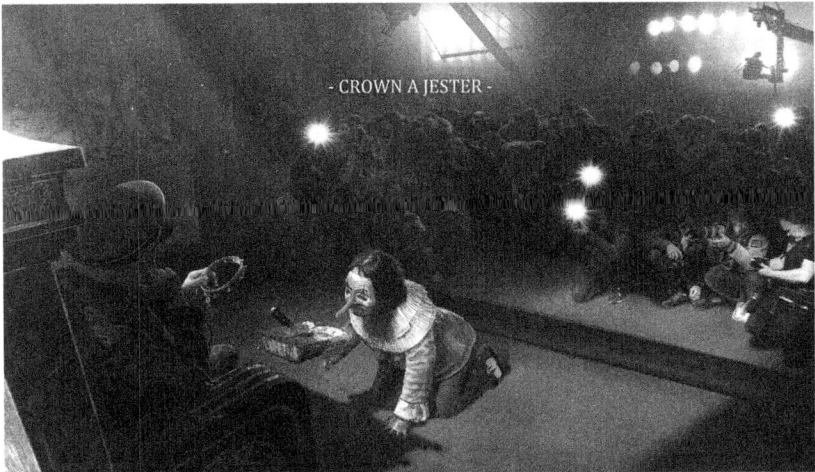

Fig. 7.1 Crown a Jester by Wuheqilin (the artist uploaded this image to Weibo with an open copyright). The artist Wuheqilin uploaded this image to Weibo on December 12, 2020, with the notice: "I reiterate that these images are completely copyright free and you may take them and use them for purposes. Feel free to cite my name or not cite my name, just don't bother sending me individual messages to seek permission"

Fang Fang and put out a public call for other martial artists to assault the writer. A partial transcript of Lei's comments provides some additional context:

> Anyone who follows what has been happening on the internet must have heard of a woman named Fang Fang. She is woman more than 50 years old from the city of Wuhan. She exploited used her so-called "tragic story" (賣慘) to describe Wuhan under lockdown during the COVID-19 outbreak in a diary. Now this diary has become a weapon used by foreigners to attack China….Right now there are all of these different fight clubs but we are lacking one that really takes the nation's hardships upon its shoulders and aims to remove the scourges who are terrorizing our society. So I would like to take this moment to call upon my fellow comrades in the martial arts world from Wuhan. As Wuhan is still under lockdown and Fang Fang has yet to leave China or Wuhan, I call upon you to condemn Fang Fang. Her words have been weaponized by foreigners to harm China leading every

Chinese person to carry a burden of unjust insults. She has caused your kindness and good-heartedness to be misunderstood by the world. History should condemn Fang Fang as a criminal. So I call on you to raise your fists in the name of justice and punish this enemy of the Chinese people. Thank you everyone![12]

It was readily evident how Lei Lei had not only been influenced by the inundation of misinformation reporting that the book had become weaponized by the West to harm China, but had fully embraced these reports as an unmitigated truth. But in the eyes of Lei Lei, this truth also functioned as a call to action. Lei Lei felt it incumbent upon himself to stand up and "in the name of justice" raise his fist to condemn Fang Fang and protect his nation. The tabloid-esque spectacle of Lei Lei's comments may illustrate a strange twist in the Fang Fang Incident's penetration into pop culture, but it also displays potential for disinformation to spin off into real-world violence. Case in point: It is likely that "the peasant" who posted big character denunciation posters near Fang Fang's residence was directly responding to Lei Lei's call.

But Lei Lei's Fang Fang chronicle was not yet over. Lei Lei had actually first come to national prominence when he accepted a challenge from mixed martial artist Xu Xiaodong 徐曉東. Xu had pledged to purge the Chinese martial arts world of all the charlatan practitioners and Lei Lei had been his first target. Before the fight Lei Lei had claimed he would be able to defeat Xu with one hand in just three seconds; instead, Lei was so brutally defeated that, beaten and bloody, he was forced to retreat from the ring after just 20 seconds. Among the responses to Lei Lei's denunciation video of Fang Fang was from none other than Xu Xiaodong. Having read Fang Fang's *Wuhan Diary*, Xu Xiaodong issued a nearly five-minute explicative-laden response to Lei Lei.[13] In his video Xu explains, "the majority of the diary is complementary and expresses hope [for the Wuhan people]; only a very small portion of the diary focusses on true criticism or complaints so I really never imagined that so many people would insult

---

[12] Lei Lei's video with the caption "Founder of Thunder God Tai Chi Lei Lei Challenges Fang Fang" (雷公太极创始人雷雷挑战方方) was uploaded to various social media platforms and widely disseminated online, including the following website: https://www.wenxuecity.com/news/2020/04/21/9383521.html.

[13] Xu Xiaodong's entire video denouncing Lei Lei is available on YouTube: https://www.youtube.com/watch?v=zc5f6dCsxa4

her." He characterized Lei's attacks on Fang Fang as "shameless" and issued a counter-appeal to Wuhan-based martial artists: "If you don't understand the truth, you will end up taking the side of the evil-doers. Open your eyes; think for yourselves, to my martial arts brothers who have a proper and just understanding of the world, please look out for Fang Fang and protect her if you are able to."[14] As Xu Xiaodong's video continued his indignation visibly grew; raising his voice, shaking his head in frustration, and pointing his finger at the camera, he declared:

> Even if Fang Fang's diary has a few sections that were not quite specific enough or had a few minor inaccuracies, those are just small issues. Overall the diary is extremely accurate and transparent. And you [Lei Lei] dare to call upon these martial artists to curse and beat this private citizen!…Fuck, for these bastards [like Lei Lei], there is no cost for patriotism. They just shout "I love my country! You're a traitor to China! You're selling us out to America!" There are a lot of fucking idiots like this in China….But let me make it perfectly clear right here: if we start seeing traces of the Cultural Revolution coming back to China, if Cultural Revolution-era practices start returning to our society, I, Xu Xiaodong, will be the first to stand up and kill you stupid motherfuckers! Fuck you all![15]

There is, in some sense, something particularly refreshing about the way Xu Xiaodong's video response provides a succinct summary of the absurdist nature of the attacks.[16] *Wuhan Diary* certainly did contain a handful of inaccuracies (almost all of which Fang Fang corrects and apologizes for in subsequent entries), but the overall thrust of the book is indeed "accurate and transparent," yet, somehow, amid the twisted and divisive world of

---

[14] Quotes from Xu Xiaodong's video are also quoted in article: "Lei Lei Wants to Beat 'Failed' Woman Writer While Xu Xiaodong Calls on the Martial World to Protect Fang Fang" (雷雷要凑败家女作家 徐晓冬吁武林:保护方方). Published on aboluowang on April, 17, 2020 https://www.aboluowang.com/2020/0417/1438226.html

[15] Quoted from Xu Xiaodong's YouTube denunciation of Lei Lei: https://www.youtube.com/watch?v=zc5f6dCsxa4

[16] It should be noted that besides standing up for Fang Fang, Xu Xiaodong has also been a public advocate for other victims of the political purge carried out in the wake of the Wuhan lockdown. In particular, former human rights lawyer and citizen journalist Chen Qiushi 陈秋實, who drew public attention after being arrested in Wuhan, made his first public appearance after being released on Xu Xiaodong's YouTube channel on September 30, 2021. https://www.youtube.com/watch?v=my8nzYX2ODA.

COVID-19 and the US-China trade war, it became politicized as a "poisonous weed" that, in the eyes of many, seemed to be the harbinger of a new era of Cultural Revolution.

It is hard for the story of Lei Lei and Xu Xiaodong not to feel like a preposterous sideshow spectacle—a Tai Chi master issuing a public denunciation and open call to arms for vigilantes to track down and "punish" a retired author who published a pandemic diary? A champion MMA fighter stepping in to call for a grassroots brigade of martial artists to protect Fang Fang? Yet these public statements from Tai Chi masters and MMA fighters were just one small corner of a complex mediasphere growing online around Fang Fang's diary, drawing in hundreds of vloggers, pop singers, artists, and public intellectuals. Collectively the handful of cases I have discussed here—diss songs, political art, and Lei Lei's calls to punish Fang Fang—are just a few of the more prominent examples of how pop culture was mobilized and weaponized against *Wuhan Diary*. These examples also attest to how a contemporary plague diary captured the attention, imagination, and, in some cases, ire of mainstream society, reverberating through the media and pop culture in unexpected ways. The deployment of pop culture was also crucial in engaging younger netizens and less politically engaged citizens in the ongoing political debate about Fang Fang. But a few months later and halfway around the world, an eerily similar dynamic has been playing out in the United States; after years of right-wing disinformation campaigns, in the summer of 2020 we started to witness the rise of militia groups using violence to stand up to the "lies" and "fake news" that had been perpetuated in the media; Dr. Fauci, the top US infectious disease specialist during the COVID-19 pandemic, began to receive death threats; and in 2021 the anti-Joe Biden rap song "Let's Go Brandon" became a viral hit. The surreal world that Lei Lei, Wuheqilin, and Bo Peep represented in China was simultaneously playing out on our own doorstep.

CHAPTER 8

Wuhan Diaries

It is curious that the diary should emerge as the primary mode trough which artists, writers, and everyday people have gravitated to in commemorating what happened in Wuhan during the early months of 2020. When we think of cultural representation of other tumultuous historical moments in recent Chinese history, from the Great Leap Forward to the Cultural Revolution and from the 1989 Tiananmen protests to the 2008 Wenchuan Earthquake, fiction, film, and documentary seem to be the mediums that most artists have employed. But somehow, the diary became *the* medium through which people will remember Wuhan 2020. Part of this is inevitably tied to the nature of the virus and how it played out. Unlike what occurred in 1989 or 2008, the novel coronavirus was not an explosive singular event, it instead played out slowly, over the course of months and not minutes or hours. And unless you or a family member was infected, this was an atrocity of the mundane, experienced by long days and seemingly endless nights of boredom, isolation, and fear as 11 million residents waited things out in their apartments. In some sense, the very private way in which the outbreak played out for millions of quarantined residents became the perfect set of circumstances for the diary to flourish. At the same time, the high level of cellphone use, internet penetration, and

M. Berry, *Translation, Disinformation, and Wuhan Diary*, https://doi.org/10.1007/978-3-031-16859-8_8

widespread adoption of social media platforms like WeChat and Weibo allowed digital diaries to proliferate during the lockdown period.[1]

Fang Fang's diary certainly also played a role in the popularity and widespread adoption of the diary format in Wuhan. Not only did the recognition of her COVID-19 chronicle become a powerful example of the literary form's power and impact, but Fang Fang also played an important role in the promotion of diary writing through her repeated calls for readers to write their own stories. She emphasized the fact that there is no "one story"; instead readers should watch CCTV and read Xinhua, but they should also read investigative reports from independent media outlets, and, most importantly, they should record their own stories.

> At the same time, I recommend that all people in Wuhan who have writing skills start recording everything they have seen, heard, experienced, and felt since January. I also hope that amateur writers also establish working groups to seek out families who lost loved ones to the coronavirus in order to help them document what their family members went through in search of treatment and what they experienced before their death. They should set up a website where all these testimonials can be uploaded and categorized for convenient searching. If possible, print versions of these testimonials published in multiple volumes would also be an important contribution. Let all of us in Wuhan leave behind a collective memory of what happened. I promise to do my part in contributing whatever help I can muster to support this cause.[2]

Through actively encouraging a sea of divergent narratives to flourish, Fang Fang is also advocating for a model of civil society where, to borrow a term from an earlier era of Chinese history, "a hundred flowers bloom and a hundred schools of thought contend." This appeal to collective witnessing can also be read as a call to arms, an attempt to foster a heteroglossia of voices to offset the singular hegemonic historical view advocated by the state. It is hard to quantify the role *Wuhan Diary* had in galvanizing other writers and bloggers to take up the pen during the early lockdown,

---

[1] For a more comprehensive overview of other lockdown diaries in Wuhan during the early phase of the COVID-19 pandemic, see Guobin Yang's monograph *The Wuhan Lockdown*. New York, Columbia University Press, 2021.

[2] Fang Fang. *Wuhan Diary: Dispatches from a Quarantined City*. New York: HarperVia, 2020. Pg. 249.

but her impact was profound, as evidenced by the large number of references to Fang Fang in the online writings of other diarists.

It wasn't long after Fang Fang's public calls for testimony that a crop of grassroots websites indeed started to pop up online. One such website, Wuhan: The Human Realm (Wuhan Renjian 武漢人間; wuhancrisis.com), featured a catalog of "emergency posts," a record of citizens calling out for help during the height of the outbreak in Wuhan. The hundreds of posts included were uploaded to social media sites from February 3, 2020, to March 14, 2020. From the posts, readers are provided with a comprehensive chronicle of the plight faced by hundreds of patients. Posts include not only basic medical information, age, and symptoms of patients, but many of the entries also include supporting documents as downloadable attachments, including CT scans, doctors' notes, and screenshots of the original social media posts. Here is an example of a fairly typical post from February 7:

> The doctor said that my grandmother has a severe infection in both lungs; she is also advanced in age so there is a real risk of pathological changes. My father also has an infection in both lungs and is now experiencing difficulty breathing. The doctor sternly told us that we need to do whatever it takes to get them both admitted to a hospital as soon as possible. I'm including my father's and grandmother's CT scans and blood results (this is my father's first CT scan, I'm at the hospital now and the second scan is at home, but the results of that scan seemed to show increased calcification in the aorta and other changes; it is really quite serious). I really can't go on waiting for someone from the district to step in to help us. Right now we are in a race against time!![3]

Reading through the hundreds of posts is a shattering experience and one cannot help but wonder how many of those patients ended getting the medical care they needed. From the number of patients documented, website users can also get a sense of the curve of the outbreak in Wuhan, with the number of posts peaking on February 5 with 252 entries before eventually dropping to double digits between February 8 and 23 and again dropping to single digits between February 24 and March 14. The website is an invaluable depository of firsthand accounts of what patients

---

[3] The original URL was https://www.wuhancrisis.com/page34/ but like so much of the documentation about the COVID-19 outbreak in Wuhan, this website has since been completely shut down.

experienced during those key crucial weeks in February and March 2020. It also provided an important record for epidemiologists and infectious disease specialists trying to understand the presentation of symptoms in early COVID-19 cases.

Humans of Wuhan (https://humansofwuhan.com) was an English-language website devoted to "everyday stories happening in Wuhan and other regions affected by the Coronavirus outbreak. Posts on the site are divided into different categories: Healthcare Providers, Patients, Reporters, Residents, and Those Who Passed Away, culling writing from a dozen different writers and platforms. And unlike the site Wuhan: The Human Realm, which focused more on cries for help and clinical presentation of patients in dire need of medical care, Humans of Wuhan was a more narrative-driven repository of stories and testimonies. According to one of the website's founders, Humans of Wuhan was not directly inspired by Fang Fang; instead, the "goal was to call for empathy from the English language readers as an effort against the anti-Chinese/Asian sentiment at that time."[4] Another portal documenting oral histories and records of Wuhan coronavirus patients is the site @the_unrecorded (未被记录的Ta们), which was started as a Twitter feed in February 2020 (https://twitter.com/the_unrecorded). According to their description, "This is an obituary page for victims of the coronavirus. Unlike the one tallied in the *New York Times*, these people do not appear in the official government tally of coronavirus victims. They had the symptoms of COVID-19 yet due to a scarcity of medical resources, their cause of death was officially listed as 'severe pneumonia,' 'infectious pneumonia,' or respiratory failure.' Because they are not included in official discourse when it comes to mourning the dead, we are needed to record and write about them. We remember so as to not repeat the same mistakes again." Collectively, these and other sites like them open up an alternative space to mourn and remember. In many ways, they are the collective fulfillment of Fang Fang's call for a "wailing web":

> ...we should really establish a website that can function as a "wailing wall"; perhaps we can call it the "wailing web." That would provide a place for mourning families to go where they could post photos, light candles, and have a good cry. Actually, it isn't just family members of the deceased who

[4] Email correspondence with webmaster of Humans of Wuhan, who wished to remain anonymous.

are crying. Everyone in the entire city of Wuhan needs a good cry; this "wailing web" could serve as a portal for people to mourn and cry for their family members, friends, and themselves. We need to release the sadness in our hearts and we need to express our grief over all the loss we have witnessed. Perhaps the website could also feature some comforting music, which might make it even better. Perhaps after we have all let out our tears and cries of mourning, we will all feel a bit better.[5]

All over internet there emerged a series of websites, social media accounts, and online portals that bore witness to what happened in Wuhan during the early months of 2020. However, like the purge of *Wuhan Diary*, as of 2022, the URLs for both The Human Realm and Humans of Wuhan are now completely shut down. While the memory of the internet, in theory, can last forever, in reality it sometimes proves even more fragile, transitory, and unreliable than human memory.

Eventually we began to see a sharp bifurcation of the *Wuhan Diary* narrative between China and the West. Internationally, *Wuhan Diary* gained an increasing amount of attention; it was translated into more than 20 different languages, it became a bestseller in Germany and other countries, and was featured in mainstream media outlets like *The New York Times, The London Times, The Guardian, The Economist, Der Spiegel,* and *Asahi Shimbun.* A small handful of other diaries also became available outside of China: excerpts from documentary filmmaker and scholar Ai Xiaoming's 艾曉明 *Wuhan Diary* appeared in the *New Left Review;*[6] feminist activist and social worker Guo Jing's 郭晶 *Wuhan Lockdown Diary* (*Wuhan fengcheng riji* 武漢封城日記) appeared in book form in Taiwan and later in an abridged English-translation online;[7] Ni Ke's 尼克 *Going Home: A Record of Taiwanese who Escaped from the Outbreak in Wuhan* (*Fanjia: Hubei Wuhan shoukun Taiwanren Fengcheng taoyi ji* 返家:湖北武漢受困台灣人封城逃疫記) was published in Taiwan by *China Times;* Bingtao Chen published *Wuhan confidentiel: D'un confinement à un autre,* a French-language memoir by an author who experienced the COVID-19 outbreak first in Wuhan and later again in Paris, comparing the radically different responses between China and Europe; and Chinese-Canadian writer Zhang Ling 張翎 published a non-fiction collection of essays in

---

[5] Fang Fang. *Wuhan Diary: Dispatches from a Quarantined City.* New York: HarperVia, 2020. Pg. 274
[6] https://newleftreview.org/issues/II122/articles/xiaoming-ai-wuhan-diary
[7] https://u.osu.edu/mclc/2020/04/27/guo-jings-wuhan-lockdown-diary/

Taiwan under the title *Panic-stricken on the Road* (*Yilu huangkong* 一路惶恐). And even more diaries, journals, and blogs proliferated on various websites and social media platforms.

However, within China, Fang Fang's *Wuhan Diary*, whose book-form Chinese-language publication had been blocked,[8] silently retreated into the background to be replaced by an army of alternative Wuhan diaries: *The Angels Diaries* (*Tianshi riji* 天使日記), a collection of 196 diary entries written by frontline medical personnel; *2020 Wuhan Diary* (*2020 Wuhan riji* 2020武漢日記), a collection of illustrations documenting the construction of the temporary hospitals built in Wuhan; *Diary of the Battle Against the Virus* (*Zhanyi riji* 戰疫日記), a collection of frontline reports from Wuhan; *Wuhan Diary of Resistance Against the Virus* (*Wuhan kangyi riji* 武漢抗疫日記), a collection of 580 short essays documenting the 76 days of the Wuhan lockdown; and *The Battle for Wuhan: Diaries of Journalists on the COVID-19 Frontline* (*Wuhan Zhanyi riji* 武汉战疫日记), a selection of articles and reports by Xinhua journalists in Wuhan. This first wave of diaries published between March and August of 2020 and other PRC publications on the Wuhan outbreak strike a very different pose than Fang Fang's *Wuhan Diary* and other accounts published internationally.

Although all of these publications are marketed and presented as "diaries," they are in fact collective accounts drawn from dozens of different authors and contributors. This is very different from the unified personal voice that comes through in the diaries of Fang Fang, Guo Jing, or Ai Xiaoming. Similarly, even the editorial credit for these publications lies not with a single individual, but rather with editorial teams and publication collectives: *Wuhan Diary of Resistance Against the Virus* is edited by "Sina Weibo Sina Reading"; *Diary of the Battle Against the Virus* is edited by "*Guangming Daily*'s Wuhan Frontline Reporting Group" 光明日報武漢一線報導組; *The Angels Diaries* is credited to "Central Radio and Television" 中央廣播電視總台中國之聲; and *The Battle for Wuhan: Diaries of Journalists on the COVID-19 Frontline* is edited by the Xinhua News Agency Wuhan frontline journalist team 新華社武漢前方報導團隊. In July 2020 Hubei People's Publishing House even launched an entire book series under the title "Diaries on the Battle Against the Virus" (*Kangyi riji xilie tushuxilie* 抗疫日記系列圖書系列), with the first two

---

[8] Many of Fang Fang's entries can still be found online and excerpts have been published in the Taiwan-based literary journal *INK*.

titles being *Diary of the Battle Against the Virus at Leishenshan Hospital* (*Leishenshan kangyi riji* 雷神山抗疫日記) by Zhao Dongfang 趙東方 and *My Temporary Hospital Diary* (*Wo de fangcang riji* 我的房艙日記) by Li Xueying 李雪穎. While these publications contain many valuable and moving accounts by medical workers, patients, volunteers, and everyday citizens in Wuhan during the outbreaks, they are also highly politicized and inundated with "positive energy." *The Battle for Wuhan: Diaries of Journalists on the COVID-19 Frontline* features a back-cover blurb by none other than Xi Jinping, and the editorial description of *Diary of the Battle Against the Virus* states:

> This book reveals an accurate account of the Chinese people's resolve to conquer the novel coronavirus under the strong leadership of the Party Central Committee with Comrade Xi Jinping at its core. The Wuhan front-line reporters went straight to the scene where they dug deep and provided a complete account of what happened. Each report contained in this book is so real, vivid, heartwarming, and moving. This book conveys to the reader firm ideals and beliefs, like "No matter what hardships we face, we shall rise up and overcome," we must face our challenges head-on and push forward, work hard and do our best to control the outbreak and ensure that economic and social development can continue as planned so as to make a positive contribution to the building of a thoroughly prosperous society. This book is our way of paying our respects to those frontline medical workers, PLA soldiers, and other comrades who stood at the front lines in this battle against the coronavirus. This book is also suitable as a study guide for party members nationwide, cadres, students from elementary school through college, and the broad masses.[9]

Obviously, this description (and other similar descriptions employed for the other books listed above) strikes a very different tone than *Wuhan Diary*. In fact, these publications can almost be read as revisionist attempts

---

[9] This description can be found on online descriptions for the book, including its listing on the popular internet bookstore Dang Dang: http://product.dangdang.com/28520119.html. The original description reads: 本书展现了中国人民在以习近平同志为核心的党中央坚强领导下坚决打赢新冠肺炎疫情的真实场景。武汉一线报道组直击一线，深度挖掘、全面阐述。每篇报道都那么真实、生动、温暖、感人。本书给读者传达了坚定的理想信念，"磨难压不垮　奋起正当时"，我们一定要迎难而上，奋力拼搏，尽力做好疫情防控和各项经济社会发展工作，为如期全面建成小康社会贡献力量。此书是向奋战在疫情防控*线的广大医务工作者、人民解放军指战员、各条战线的同志们*好的敬意。此书适合作为全国广大党员、干部、人民群众、大中小学生的参考学习读物。

to redress the "errors" of Fang Fang. Everything the ultra-leftists criticized *Wuhan Diary* for—a lack of patriotism, not enough attention to grand acts like the construction of the Huoshenshan 火神山醫院 and Leishenshan Hospitals 雷神山醫院 and the "victory" over the virus, and an individual perspective relying upon reports from friends and the internet that was perceived as "hearsay," and accused of "spreading rumors"— is amended in the pages of these officially sanctioned accounts. Instead of Fang Fang's view from her apartment, there is an overwhelming attention to "the front line," grand national narratives that Fang Fang eschewed for depictions of the everyday are here refocused, the individual is firmly repositioned within a sweeping collective narrative of national struggle and sacrifice, the unofficial nature of Fang Fang's blog is replaced with government-sanctioned narratives curated by official news outlets, and where Fang Fang's diary was transformed into a "poisonous weed," these books are to be seen as "study guides" for all of society. While official publication of Fang Fang's diary was suppressed, these official Wuhan diaries not only inundated the market, but also appeared in a sophisticated high-tech form: for instance, *2020 Wuhan Diary* and *The Battle for Wuhan: Diaries of Journalists on the COVID-19 Frontline* were among several publications in this category that featured dozens of embedded QR codes, which linked to various online content including news articles, documentaries, and even music videos. The embedded QR codes link the experience of reading about COVID-19 to the lived experience of the lockdown in China, where scanning health QR codes became an integral part of people's daily lives in post-COVID-19 China; at the same time, it could be argued that the QR codes embedded into the text further accentuate and legitimize the scientific truth and verifiable facts behind the diary entries. By embedding QR codes into these books about the Wuhan outbreak, a symbiosis is created between daily acts and sentiments of health and safety and these officially sanctioned print/digital narratives of frontline healthcare workers. I would argue that this synthesis works on a deep psychological level: scanning heath QR codes is a key step to ensure the safety of everyday citizens and the act of scanning itself creates an instantaneous sense of psychological security and relief, just as scanning QR codes from these publications reveals the correct narrative, the "good story" of sacrifice and heroism that paved the way for China to control the virus. The discrepancy between the absence of the original *Wuhan Diary*, which of course made its first appearance as a purely online phenomenon, and this new high-tech literary form which melded a traditional reading experience with online engagement seemed to further accentuate the rift between Fang Fang's now "obsolete" diary and these new positive, accurate, firsthand accounts that were now even taking on a futuristic form that mirrored and reinforced this new technological side of people's daily lives.

If the difference wasn't already clear enough, the state tabloid the *Global Times* further emphasized the fundamental rift between Fang Fang's account and that of state-approved narratives. A November 8, 2020, article promoting a new "Wuhan diary" entitled *Wuhan Girl: A Nian's Diary* (*Wuhan nuhai: A Nian riji* 武漢女孩:阿念日記) opened with the following comparison:

> "Is this another 'Wuhan Diary' like Fang Fang's?" This is the question some Chinese netizens posed after young woman Wu Shangzhe 吳尚哲, also known as A Nian 阿念, published her personal story about what her family experienced in Wuhan, Central China's Hubei Province, during the world's strictest COVID-19 lockdown.
>
> However, compared to the controversy stirred by *Wuhan Diary*, which took a critical stance toward the lockdown, the book *Wuhan Girl A Nian Diary* projects warmth, empathy and optimism, giving hope to many Chinese readers wrestling with the bitterness of life.[10]

Written by a screenwriter Wu Shangzhe, who suffered from COVID-19 during the early outbreak in Wuhan and lost her grandmother to the virus, *Wuhan Girl: A Nian's Diary* was heavily promoted by state media outlets. The book jacket displayed the endorsements of the *People's Daily*, Xinhua News, and CCTV News alongside various luminaries from the Chinese cultural world. The description above lays bare the seemingly now "official verdict" on *Wuhan Diary*, which is condemned for its "critical stance" in favor of narratives of "warmth, empathy and optimism." Around the same time as *Wuhan Girl: A Nian's Diary* was gaining accolades in the Chinese press, the opera *Angel's Diary*, a tribute to medical workers fighting on the front lines of the pandemic, also premiered in Wuhan to get critical acclaim. What is interesting is that, more than eight months after the attacks on *Wuhan Diary*, official Chinese narratives about the Wuhan outbreak were still being framed against Fang Fang's account. Curious

---

[10] Chen Xi. "'Wuhan Girl A Nian Diary'—young Chinese woman's tough experience during COVID-19 lockdown moves readers" November 6, 2020. *The Global Times*. https://www.globaltimes.cn/content/1205924.shtml

how Fang Fang's account could be simultaneously rendered invisible, while driving how so much of other "official narratives" were shaped.[11] Earlier, I suggested in tongue-and-cheek fashion that perhaps *Wuhan Diary* could not be accepted as a true "diary" by her detractors because it deviated too far from the patriotic model of *The Diary of Lei Feng*—the original model of what a politically correct, "positive energy" diary should be. Just a few months later, an entire genre of Wuhan diaries would arise that would be thoroughly imbued with the revolutionary fervor of Lei Feng. In the months following the attack on Fang Fang's book, more and more of these new "Wuhan diaries" inundated the Chinese market—by the end of 2020 there was well over a dozen in print, none of them written by Fang Fang. Instead, joining *Wuhan Girl* and the various diaries chronicling the "battle against the virus," there were *Dr. Zha's Diary of Fighting COVID-19* (*Zha yisheng yuan'e riji* 查醫生援鄂日記), which also published in English translation; *Wuhan! Wuhan! A Diary of Wuhan's Struggle Against the Virus* (*Wuhan! Wuhan! Wuhan kangyi riji* 武漢!武漢!武漢抗疫日記); *White Notebook* (*Baise jishibo* 白色記事薄); *Confidence Comes from Effectiveness: A Foreigner's Wuhan Diary* (*Jianding: Yige waiguoren de Wuhan riji* 堅定:一個外國人的武漢日記), written by Adham Sayed, a Lebanese student studying in Wuhan who described his diary as an effort to "protect the truth like a soldier"; and even children's books like *Little Kitty's Diary: The Kitty with a Facemask* (*Xiaomao riji: dai kouzhao de mao* 小貓日記:戴口罩的貓), which told the story of the lockdown from a kitten's perspective, and *A Record of San Mao's Fight Against the Virus*

---

[11]A similar phenomenon can be observed in the case of the 1937 Nanjing Massacre. During the mid-1980s, in the wake of a series of public denials made by prominent Japanese politicians and public figures, the Chinese response was the production of a massive number of films, documentaries, non-fiction books, diaries, and novels all focusing on the issue of "evidence" (*zhengju* 證據) and "testimony" (*jianzheng* 見證). In this case, Chinese cultural discourse around the Nanjing Massacre in the 1980s was shaped, in large part, by a few isolated of Japanese denial and a massive nationalistic thrust to provide "evidence" to refute those claims. In the case of the 2020 Wuhan outbreak, a similar dynamic can be observed, where massive numbers of books, documentaries, stage plays, and television dramas have been produced to refute and correct the "ideological errors" of *Wuhan Diary* while, simultaneously, borrowing from Fang Fang's "diary" format.

(*San Mao kangyi ji* 三毛抗疫記), which featured one of China's most beloved cartoon icons doing his part to fight COVID-19.[12]

As the number of these diaries proliferated, so too did official state media's efforts to promote these works and, in the process, further discredit Fang Fang. Many of these state-endorsed diaries were released in both Chinese-language and English-language editions. One case in point occurred on May 14, 2021, when Spokesperson for the Ministry of Foreign Affairs of the People's Republic of China Zhao Lijian 趙立堅 celebrated the English-language publication of Adham Sayed's account, *Confidence Comes from Effectiveness: A Foreigner's Wuhan Diary*, with the following tweet:

> The real #Wuhan Diary, Confidence Comes from Effectiveness: A Foreigner's Wuhan Diary, was translated from #Arabic into #English.[13]

Without mentioning Fang Fang by name, Zhao's emphasis of Sayed's account as "the real #Wuhan Diary" is a clear endorsement of the numerous allegations against Fang Fang as someone that was indeed engaged in peddling lies and spreading disinformation. The tweet was embedded with a link to a *China Daily* article about the book's publication, but, more significantly, it stood out for being one of the few high-level political figures in China to address *Wuhan Diary*, albeit indirectly via an endorsement of one of the clone diaries produced to take its place. The decision to single out and promote Sayad's account as a "foreigner" was no doubt

---

[12] Besides the inundation of official diary format books on the Wuhan outbreak, a parallel group of official narratives also appeared in China that narratized the event as a "heroic battle," often embellishing vocabulary and imagery related to war. This is a theme also evident in many of the official Wuhan diary-style narratives, but it is even further embellished in such books as *The Hero: Chinese Communist Party Members on the Front Lines of the Battle Against COVID-19* (*Gongchandangyuan zai kangyi yixian* 共產黨員在抗疫一線), *China Battles the Virus* (*Zhanyi Zhongguo* 戰疫中國), *Striking the Virus: We Are Taking Action* (*Kangji yiqing: Women zai xingdong* 抗擊疫情：我們在行動), *Academicians Fighting the Virus* (*Yuanshi zhanyi* 院士戰疫), *The Economic Battle Against the Virus* (*Jingji zhanyi* 經濟戰疫), *A Record of Heroes Against the Virus* (*Kangyi yingxiong pu* 抗疫英雄譜), *The Shield of Battle Against the Virus* (*Zhanyi zhi dun* 戰疫之盾), *Salute the Heroes* (*Zhijing yingxiong* 致敬英雄), and *The People's Battle Against the Virus* (*Renmin zhanyi* 人民戰疫). All of these titles speak to the robust narrative being created in China where the COVID-19 outbreak and response were framed with powerful wartime narrative tropes about sacrifice, heroism, selflessness, and nationalism.

[13] Lijian Zhao @zlj517 tweet posted on May 14, 2021. https://twitter.com/zlj517/status/1393147855238402054

an attempt to lend an extra layer of objective truth to his diary. However, it is telling that among the long comments thread following Zhao Lijian's tweet, there are few messages actually engaging with Adam Sayed's book, and, instead, many of the messages are dominated by attacks on Fang Fang such as "Fang Fang, show yourself and take your beating!" and "Fang Fang, I heard ny friend say this account is the real thing."[14]

A similar bifurcation of Wuhan narratives can also be seen in other narrative accounts, such as documentary filmmaking, which alongside the diary format has emerged as one of the most powerful mediums for portraying the pandemic. In China, a series of documentaries highlighting the official narrative were quickly produced. These include documentary serials produced by state-run entities like CCTV and include *City of Heroes* (*Yingxiong zhi cheng* 英雄之城), *Wuhan: A Diary of My Battle Against the "Virus"* (*Wuhan: Wo de zhan "yi" riji* 武漢:我的戰"疫"日記), and *Record of China's Battle Against the Virus* (*Zhongguo zhanyi lu* 中國戰疫錄). Notice the ubiquitous use of language that frames COVID-19 through the lens of a military operation in almost all of the official narratives, repeatedly emphasizing words like "heroes" and "battle." At the same time, we have seen an increasing number of independently produced documentaries about Wuhan circulating internationally, such as Ai Weiwei's 艾未未 *Coronation* (*Jiamian* 加冕), Hao Wu's *76 Days* (*76 tian* 76天), and Nanfu Wang's *In the Same Breath*. And then there are films caught in the middle, like Yung Chang's *Wuhan Wuhan* (武漢 武漢); its US debut at DOC NYC was cancelled just a few weeks before its premiere for "technical reasons," a euphemistic phrase that has been used to explain the cancellation of numerous Chinese films at various festivals in recent years for "political reasons." It was only six months later in late April 2021 that *Wuhan Wuhan* would receive a belated release at Hot Docs. Like the fractured way in which the diary narratives have circulated, we are seeing an identical trend occurring in the realm of documentary film.

But how do we account for this split? Part of this goes back to David Der-wei Wang's earlier comments on the political imperative to "tell the good China story." When it comes to the COVID-19 outbreak, Wang writes:

[14] Ibid.

…in the midst of the coronavirus outbreak in 2020, Xi called on Chinese citizens to "tell the good China story of fighting the epidemic." Some did not need Xi's prompting. Li Wenliang (1986–2020), a medical whistle-blower, attempted to warn the authorities about the coming crisis in late 2019 and was punished for spreading what was called a rumor. Li contracted the virus from a patient and died three days after Xi's call for a good story; he was later officially honored as a "martyr." Was Li's a good story?[15]

Li Wenliang's early attempt to notify colleagues about the coronavirus was certainly interpreted by local authorities as "the wrong story." He was reprimanded and forced to sign a confession; but after the unprecedented public outcry in the wake of his death, Li was posthumously rehabilitated, named a "martyr," and in official discourse his efforts have now became a crucial page in the "good story." In the case of Fang Fang, things went in the opposite direction. Fang Fang was, after all, a writer with close ties to the official state cultural apparatus and had garnered tens of millions of loyal readers for her account of the coronavirus outbreak. Perhaps Fang Fang's *Wuhan Diary* started out as a "good story," that is, until the powers that be deemed it wasn't. And once the book had been thoroughly suppressed and subjected to ample doses of criticism and attacks, new "good stories" were needed to take its place. Just as China adopted a "Zero COVID" stance in terms of public health policy, so too it simultaneously implemented a zero tolerance policy when it came to narratives about COVID-19 that deviated from the official playbook. The inundation of "official Wuhan diaries" or "good diaries" can also be seen as an illustration of what Margaret E. Roberts has described as flooding, "pushing particular types of information to the top of the pyramid in order to de-emphasize others."[16] This sea of "official Wuhan diaries" was a conscious attempt to fill the void of Fang Fang's absence, to replace her "heretical" *Wuhan Diary* with a new hegemonic master narrative. Looked at collectively, it was a stunning display of mass mobilization of writers, editors, and publishers; the dozens of alternative Wuhan diaries that appeared within one year of the Wuhan lockdown (many of which written in a format eerily reminiscent to that of Fang Fang) speak to the unprecedented efforts expended to displace Fang Fang's original narrative with an entire genre of "proper" and "correct" alternatives. The Hubei People's Publishing House even described its motivation in releasing

---

[15] David Der-wei Wang. *Why Fiction Matters in Contemporary China*, pg. 176.
[16] Roberts, Margaret E. *Censored: Distraction and Diversion Inside China's Great Firewall.* Princeton: Princeton University Press, 2018. Pg. 43

a book series devoted to pandemic diaries as aiming to "tell the *good story* of the battle against the virus and promote the spirit of resistance against the virus."[17] This reconstituted narrative, a "positive energy" or *zheng nengli-ang* 正能量 narrative, if you will, was brimming with hope and tears, sacrifice and perseverance, and ultimately victory and gratitude. The speed at which this transference took place displays just how manipulative and effective the machinery of propaganda can be, especially as it is now aided by the full power of the internet. At the same time, the process also seems to attest to just how fickle public whims can be, when manipulated by a deluge of disinformation and fake news. Of course, telling the "good China story" is also a tale of translation. How is the history unfolding before our eyes translated into a story? But we must ask, as that narrative is translated, what gets played down, what gets amplified and embellished, and what gets forgotten? How did the tone of the story transform so radically from fear, uncertainty, anger, and helplessness to jubilation, celebration, national pride, and victory? The *good story* of the COVID-19 outbreak in Wuhan was a project in which master narratives were manufactured through editorial manipulation and selective translation.

Telling the good China story is also about cultural power—the power to shape narratives and control discourse and the power to silence voices that diverge from the correct story. The manipulation of the good story not only impacts how we perceive COVID-19 today, but also anticipates how the history of the outbreak will be preserved for the future. The inundation of the alternative Wuhan diaries not only supplants Fang Fang's narrative, but effectively establishes what the "true history" will be moving forward. As Zheng Wang has observed: "Choosing what to remember and what to forget is not a simple sorting process for history education. Historical memory is more than an understanding of history. How the government defines history is a deeply political issue that is closely related to the legitimacy of the government and rightly shapes the national identity of China."[18] But we should also realize that the successful control of the COVID-19 outbreak in China is also tied to a parallel display of

---

[17] "Hubei People's Publishing House Rolls Out a Community Events to Promote its 'Diaries on the Battle Against the Virus Book Series'" ("Hubei renmin chubanshe qidong 'Kangyi riji xilie tushuxilie shequ xuanchuan huodong'" 湖北人民出版社啟動抗疫日記系列圖書系列社區宣傳活動) July 27, 2020. (no author cited). https://www.sohu.com/a/410000735_207067

[18] Wang, Zheng. *Never Forget National Humiliation: Historical Memory in Chinese Politics and Foreign Relations.* New York: Columbia University Press, 2012. Pg. 6.

political power: the power to enforce strict quarantines and travel restrictions and implement tracking, tracing, and testing mechanisms. We would be remiss to not ponder and interrogate the interrelations between the way power has been wielded in these two cases. In particular, we should reflect on the ways in which the success of the latter display of power (to control COVID-19) provided additional political justification for efforts to further shape cultural discourse and curb open speech.

One of the stranger and more perverse and uncanny examples to emerge from the "Wuhan Diary genre" was the appearance of "American Diary." The diary was posted daily as a blog on Weibo by Yam Bear Six (Diguaxiong laoliu 地瓜熊老六), a comic book artist and registered Weibo VIP user with more than six million followers who identifies himself as "Captain of the Patriot Brigade" (愛國小分隊隊長) at the end of each diary entry. As of March 10, 2022, Yam Bear Six's "American Diary" has already published 582 entries on Weibo, nearly 10 times the volume of Fang Fang's original diary which it parodies. Primarily aimed at revealing the failure of US policy and leadership in the wake of the coronavirus outbreak, the entries satirically employ the basic structure of Fang Fang's *Wuhan Diary*, embellishing the most commonly employed criticisms of the book through parody. For instance, alluding to the repeated claims that Fang Fang's diary is nothing but hearsay composed of secondary accounts the author "heard from friends," "American Diary" frequently features passages like: "Today my friend from a US hospital told me, my American friend Old Donald has continued sending out tweets from the hospital: 'STOCK MARKET HIGHS! VOTE!'..."[19] or "Today a friend of mine from the White House told me that the White House online store is now selling commemorative coins celebrating Old Donald's victory over the coronavirus, they are on sale for 100 USD each and it is a limited edition pressing of only 2500 coins. The first 1000 customers will receive a complimentary presidential facemask the same as the president's. My American friend Old Donald is quite the industrious little money maker; not only does he reap in the votes, but he also rakes in the cash—two birds with one stone!"[20]

[19] Yam Bear Six 地瓜熊老六. "American Diary 191: 2020 seems to be a big glorious year for FF; but actually it has been a shameless year of lament" ("Meiguo riji 191: 2020 maosi FF de fengguang danian, shize gengshi ta de wuchi ainian" 美國日記191:2020貌似FF的風光大年，實則更是她的無恥哀年) October, 5, 2020 on Weibo: https://weibo.com/ttarticle/p/show?id=2309404556812870353181#_0
[20] Ibid.

Naturally, Yam Bear Six's parody diary did not just employ Fang Fang's diary form and attempt to turn earlier criticisms of the diary into a mockery, "American Diary" also used its influential platform to continue launching targeted attacks on Fang Fang herself. For instance, the same 2000-character entry from October 5, 2020, Yam Bear Six ends as follows:

> In conclusion, I would like to say: 2020 seems to be a big glorious year for Fang Fang; she has published her big Eight-Nation Diary 八國日記, she has won the praises of the White House, but actually these things are all testament to what has been a shameless year of lament. That's because she is indeed wrong. And her wrongs have now been translated by the thugs in America and other foreign countries as a record to show the world. But I don't believe for one second that Fang Fang will be able to continue living her carefree life outside the confines of the law. One day, Fang Fang will outlive her usefulness and be heartlessly abandoned by her master![21]

The "Eight-Nation Diary" is an allusion to the Eight-Nation Alliance that suppressed the Boxer Rebellion during the Qing dynasty—a military action that resulted in the loss of priceless Chinese relics and the destruction of many important cultural sites, like the Old Summer Palace. The actions are still regarded today as a key moment in China's "century of humiliation" at the hands of Western powers, and here, Fang Fang's diary is positioned as an extension of that legacy of Western aggression against China. "Praises of the White House" is a reference to a Chinese-language speech delivered on May 4, 2020, by then Deputy National Security Advisor Matt Pottinger at the Miller Center at the University of Virginia, where he briefly mentions Fang Fang alongside a group of individuals he recognizes for their "big acts of moral and physical courage."[22] However, in the eyes of average Chinese netizens, this rhetoric goes a long way in cementing the relationship between Fang Fang's diary and international anti-China conspiracies. Yam Bear's attacks on *Wuhan Diary* would continue unfettered, growing in popularity and becoming bolder and

[21] Ibid.
[22] The remarks here cited were originally delivered in Chinese by Matthew Pottinger to mark the anniversary of the May Fourth Movement. An English translation of his full speech "Remarks by Deputy National Security Advisor Matt Pottinger to the Miller Center at the University of Virginia" is available in text format here: https://www.whitehouse.gov/briefings-statements/remarks-deputy-national-security-advisor-matt-pottinger-miller-center-university-virginia/ or in video format here https://www.youtube.com/watch?v=dp5h6n6fbUg.

more egregious in their conspiratorial claims over time. In episode 296 of his *American Diary*, Yam Bear Six would further embellish his claims linking Fang Fang's diary to the Eight-Nation Alliance's aggression against China more than a century earlier:

> Finally, I want to say: A long time ago the Eight Nation Alliance invaded China; although there is no Eight Nation Alliance that would dare to invade China today, they can still publish Fang Fang's Diary! They can still award Fang Fang all kinds of literary prizes! And they can foster many more Fang Fangs! In the past, the Eight Nation Alliance used their guns and cannons to slaughter the Chinese people, but now they use the power of discourse to give the Chinese people a "soft burial!" And so we must protect ourselves against the Eight Nation Alliance's guns, but we must be even more vigilant against their literary running dogs who use the power of discourse to launch clandestine attacks against China!![23]

These types of anti-Fang Fang narratives and commentaries inundate "American Diary," and, if there is indeed a new genre of "Wuhan diaries" that has emerged in the PRC, this is the underbelly. It also played out alongside a broader online critical discourse in China that called for the production of various other diaries—such as "New York Diary" or "Los Angeles Diary"—that were meant to undermine Fang Fang's account and further highlight US missteps.[24] Concept cover images for *New York Diary: Dispatches from the USA* depicting a design reminiscent of the HarperVia cover of *Wuhan Diary* with a grim reaper replacing the globe also widely circulated on Chinese social media. Meanwhile, "American Diary" reveals a curious and likely unprecedented phenomenon whereby the parody is now more expansive and, by 2022, was likely more widely circulated than the

[23] Yam Bear Six 地瓜熊老六. "American Diary 296: The power of discourse is much more destructive than an atomic bomb" ("Meiguo riji 296: Huayuquan bi yuanzidan de shashangxing gengda" 美國日記296：話語權比原子彈的殺傷性更大) January 26, 2021 on Weibo: https://weibo.com/ttarticle/p/show?id=2309404597759704432707#_0

[24] Among the many personal attacks I received as the translator, one of the most frequent and consistent was the call for me to write my own "American diary" to reveal the failure of US government in controlling COVID-19. Other iterations called for me to translate Yam Bear Six's American Diary into English.

now suppressed original.[25] While government media and publishing organizations like Xinhua News Agency publish "official accounts" that are suitable as "study guides," unofficial nationalist diaries like Yam Bear Six's "American Diary" do the real dirty work, continuing the protracted campaign to mock, undercut, and further demonize Fang Fang's account. And true to its name, over the course of its hundreds of entries, "American Diary" has also grown beyond a parody of *Wuhan Diary* and into a larger platform for attacking and mocking the United States and its policies.

In the wake of the suppression of *Wuhan Diary* within China, two new narratives have emerged, each split along geopolitical lines. In the West, the book is lauded by major media outlets; portions of the narrative which criticize the Chinese response are often emphasized, but even more prominently, they single out Fang Fang as a voice of audacious courage. Reviews of the book frequently feature passages like "This book is most scorching in Fang Fang's calls to hold to account the leaders who downgraded and minimized the virus, wasting nearly three weeks and allowing it to seep into the world at large. She rallies around this topic like Henry V pacing the floorboards before the Battle of Agincourt. She may live meekly during the lockdown, but she writes bold sentences."[26] Meanwhile in China, official media outlets like the *Global Times* featured almost universally negative coverage, with headlines like "Fang Fang and her followers criticized for weaponizing netizen's post to create biased narrative," "Fans disappointed as Wuhan Diary's overseas publication 'gives ammunition to antagonist forces,'" and "Some Chinese intellectuals hold distorted values, represented by Fang Fang." This bifurcation of the book's reception is perhaps most clearly presented in the book's Amazon reader reviews, which have been split in half between five-star genuine reader reviews and one-star troll reviews, which parrot criticisms on Weibo regarding the book's authenticity and claim it is a book of lies. The massive numbers of trolls mobilized to *chuzheng* or embark on an international campaign to discredit the book's reputation abroad attest to the transpacific dimension

---

[25] In some ways, this case is similar to online fan fiction that expands the narratives of popular novels, such as the case of Baoshu's literary expansions of Liu Cixin's science fiction world. In this case, however, Yam Bear Six's work is the antithesis of "fan" fiction and should be categorized as detractor fiction or hate fiction.

[26] Garner, Dwight. "'Wuhan Diary' offers an angry and eerie view from inside quarantine." New York Times, May 21, 2020. https://www.pilotonline.com/entertainment/books/vp-db-book-wuhan-diary-fang-fang-review-052420-20200521-jqliwdybibhl7ph4m7aa4sowye-story.html

of the attacks. Of course, online disinformation campaigns are global by the very nature of the internet and the platforms through which they are carried out; however, most online campaigns targeting Chinese intellectuals and writers have been relegated primarily to the Chinese-language cyber-sphere. In the case of *Wuhan Diary*, while changing the tenor of the discourse within China was clearly a primary objective, discrediting the book globally was also an important goal, as evidenced by review bombing of the book on international websites (like Amazon.com) and taking active measures to suppress the publication of the book abroad.

It was in the 1960s that Stanley Fish and other literary critics introduced us to literary response theory and the concept that the meaning of literary texts is not fixed, but rather repeatedly given new meaning through the interpretation of different groups of readers. Nowhere has that lesson be illustrated so powerfully than in the case of Fang Fang's *Wuhan Diary* where the book's meaning continually transformed in real time alongside the ebbs and flows of Sino-US tensions and the spread of the virus itself. Along the way, the book became a literary Rorschach test, becoming what different groups of readers needed it to be in order to serve different political interests.

As the diary's reception is split, so too is the very notion of what a "Wuhan Diary" is—with Fang Fang's *Wuhan Diary* and other "nonofficial" accounts widely circulating internationally while "official" government-sanctioned diaries have taken over the narrative within China. Through this tale of two diaries we also witness the radical bifurcation of the internet and online discourse between China and the rest of the world.[27] This is a trend that is further exacerbated by the impact of fake news and disinformation campaigns. This bifurcation began slowly; I remember more than a decade ago when YouTube was first banned in China, in order to share music clips with friends in China, I instead

---

[27] While the bifurcation of publicly voiced discourse was quite stark, as Jinquan Yu, Binghan Zheng, and Lu Shao have rightly pointed out, besides positive and negative responses to *Wuhan Diary*, another important facet were "neutral" responses: "There also existed a group of readers who adopted a relatively neutral line. Based on their analysis of both the critical and supportive voices with regard to the English translation of Fang Fang's diary in the US, they tended to support its translation into English with, however, the condition of a need to clarify and revise some of its contents to ensure its authenticity." See Jinquan Yu, Binghan Zheng & Lu Shao. "Who has the final say? English translation of online lockdown writing *Wuhan Diary*" in *Perspectives: Studies in Translation Theory and Practice*. Routledge. Published online May 26, 2021. Pg. 5.

resorted to Xiami Music, a local Chinese music streaming site, but within a year Xiami started placing restrictions on accessing the site's content from outside of China. Other sites quickly followed suit. As China one by one restricted the most popular online platforms in the West (YouTube, Facebook, Google, Netflix, Twitter, etc.), full access to the Chinese internet from abroad also started to get more complicated; many websites require a local Chinese telephone number to register or feature content unable to be downloaded or played outside of China. In 2020, as the Trump administration attempted to ban Chinese platforms like WeChat and TikTok from app stores in the United States, we found ourselves facing an increasingly dangerous situation wherein both the United States and China were each locking themselves away in their own self-contained media spheres.[28]

As tensions between China and the United States intensify, one of the chief problems is a fundamental lack of mutual understanding. Even with open lines of communication and open access to online platforms, there is an immense cultural gap to bridge, but when those lines of communication are shut down and platforms are closed, each side is left with an increasingly stilted perspective, a virtual echo chamber. We have each become the proverbial "frog in the well." China and the Unites States each tell their own "good story," usually at the expense of the other, and, in the end, the citizens on both sides end up with a worldview that is one-sided and impoverished. The bifurcation of *Wuhan Diary* is but one small example of how these parallel narratives are constructed and perpetuated through online media, digital culture, and even national policies.

---

[28] Indeed, another frequent comment I was subjected to during the attacks was "Get off Weibo!" as if foreigners had no place on the platform.

CHAPTER 9

The Strange

When you open the Weibo app on your phone, the first image to pop up is an advertisement. It only lingers on the screen for a few seconds before automatically delivering you to the platform content, unless you first click the "skip ad" button. The advertisements feature obligatory images of beautiful young models and actors, like Yang Mi 楊冪 and Lu Han 鹿晗, who are usually selling some form of luxury item, from cosmetics and luxury handbags to glasses and perfume. After using Weibo for nearly a decade, I never gave a second thought to those fleeting glossy images of overly photoshopped glamour and beauty, but at some point in mid-April of 2020, those images began to make me sick. I couldn't help but be struck by the dissonance between the perfectly idealized, sanitized, and controlled images of a manicured consumerist utopia inhabited by ideals of bodily perfection, sexual allure, and 1% lifestyle luxury and the world that lurked just beyond that façade. For just as the advertisement window would automatically close, what would inevitably be waiting for me on the other side were hundreds of new messages and posts, the majority of which were riddled with threats, curses, and slanderous lies.

As I translated Fang Fang's diary, there were many experiences imbued with a sense of the strange and uncanny. My own life became fractured in different ways: between my "normal life" in late February when I began translating *Wuhan Diary* to life under lockdown just a few weeks later; between my quotidian everyday routine (including supervising my two elementary school-age children's online classes, teaching my own online classes for UCLA, and regular household chores) and the surreal online world of the "Fang Fang Incident," which I had somehow become deeply embroiled in; and between Fang Fang's experience of life under lockdown in Wuhan and my own experience under lockdown in Los Angeles. As time went by, my own experience seemed to echo Fang Fang's in uncanny ways: she began writing a quarantine diary, a month later I started translating one; Wuhan was lockdown in late January, Los Angeles followed in early March; Fang Fang was targeted by the online trolls, and so was I. It also felt as if I was simultaneously navigating different temporalities: I was here in the present, translating events that took place just one month in the past that seemed, strangely enough, to foretell our collective future. Somehow, those few short seconds going from glossy ads on Weibo to vicious attacks seemed to capture the dissonance, disconnect, and fracture that I had been living in throughout my time translating *Wuhan Diary*.

Those moments of dissonance and the strange continued to punctuate my life over the next several months as I translated *Wuhan Diary* and began to live amid the fallout that ensued. The first wave came via the thousands of Weibo attacks. After the controversy surrounding the book's title and online book description lit up Weibo, another unusual phenomena were the aforementioned Chinese trolls that started to log onto Amazon.com in the United States and bomb the book with one-star reviews. Having followed publications on Chinese literature and culture for my entire career, this is something I had never before witnessed. Not even so-called dissident writers like Liu Xiaobo, Liao Yiwu 廖亦武, or Wei Jingsheng 魏京生 had their books attacked in this manner. A few samples of the one-star Amazon reviews of *Wuhan Diary*:

> "So pathetic,"
> "An opportunistic attempt to gain fame and money out of the pandemic situation,"
> "Her diary are composed mostly of heresy and lack any concrete evidence.... Also, one has to wonder how her book came out so quickly in the US and Europe, at the same time or before it was published in China. Fang doesn't speak English or German and yet somehow it was "translated" almost instantaneously and made it to the book stand in the west, 2 months after Wuhan's reopening. Anyone in the book publishing industry will tell you that's an impossible speed without premeditation. Premeditation... Makes one wonder if this wasn't simply a constructed, coordinated effort with anti-Chinese forces in the west intent on smearing China."

"All the things are from third person events and none of this is real. As a Wuhan doctor, I have seen most of the events but in this book, I never heard about anything that occurs here. Everything that fang fang said isn't true and is fake. Not everything of course but most are fake and some things are so warped and written under the authors desire"

"All I want to say is that This book does not deserve the name "Wu Han Diary".
It only stands for the author, not for Wuhan people.
I have some questions to the author:
Don't you feel shame when you build your stage on other people's bones and blood?
Don't you feel guilty when you use human sympathy to shine your own "glory"?
Don't you ever feel disgrace when you want to represent Wuhan people while you did nothing for them?
You were living in your mansion typing your book while people were fighting and struggling in the hospitals and homes. And now you want to sell this stories and get money and reputations back?

As that author said, same words to herself
"who do you think you are?"
You were not even a warrior, not even a part of them, and you want to tell others a world that you've never been to?
If you want to write a Wuhan Diary,
Go back to school again, learn how to cite, learn to find data, learn truth."[1]

Controlling information, even manipulating film and book reviews/ratings, is not uncommon in China, but this is one of the rare cases where trolls were motivated to "hop the fence" or "go on a crusade" (*chuzheng* 出征) and attempt to do whatever possible to compromise the influence and credibility of the publication abroad. In recent years, it has become increasingly common for prominent Chinese political figures (like Zhao Lijian, deputy director of the Chinese Ministry of Foreign Affairs Information Department) and media pundits (like Hu Xijin 胡錫進, editor-in-chief of the *Global Times*) to utilize international social media platforms banned in China (like Twitter) to promote government

---

[1] All quoted from Amazon Customer Reviews of *Wuhan Diary*. https://www.amazon. com/Wuhan-Diary-Dispatches-Quarantined-City-ebook/product-reviews/B086JXGZFB/ ref=cm_cr_dp_d_show_all_btm?ie=UTF8&reviewerType=all_reviews

positions. Then in 2016, the Diba Expedition 帝吧出征 to Facebook, in which Chinese trolls used VPNs to launch nationalist attacks on targeted Facebook pages, signaled a major shift in how Chinese cyber-attack campaigns are waged. The "event created shock waves to public opinion about the shape and strength of China's so-called Internet nationalism."[2] But this was something different. I read the attempts to discredit *Wuhan Diary* not only within China, but also through international "review-bombing" on sites like Amazon as a concerted effort to undermine and discredit the book globally. Of course, one can never pinpoint exactly where the reviews were geographically generated from, but *Wuhan Diary* was flooded with review after review that simply parroted the main talking points against the book that had been circulating in Chinese social media posts, articles, and Weibo during the previous months. In another strange twist, screenshots of some of these one-star reviews on Amazon were then uploaded to Weibo (with Chinese translations) to "prove" how poorly the book was being received internationally.

And then it just got weirder. On April 25, 2020, still during the height of the online attacks, I received a "fan email" from someone named "Alex Penis." Mr. Penis expressed his admiration for my translation and offered to share a cache of related documents labeled "Wuhan's Cries for Help," which was attached as a massive 17.5 MB Word file. I wasn't quite sure that I was quite ready to receive "Wuhan's Cries for Help" from Mr. Penis ... I remembered that the very first Amazon review of *Wuhan Diary* that had been uploaded ten days earlier, on April 15, was a one-star troll attack by a user named none other than "Alex." Two days before that, on April 13, a user named "Alex's Viewpoint" uploaded a nearly 18-minute video to YouTube entitled "What is Fangfang diary? Wuhan Diary? It is a fiction not a diary from anti-China forces."[3] Were all of these coming from the same person? In the meantime, Mr. Penis was getting restless and emailed me a second time. Just out of curiosity, I googled Alex Penis' email address but the only results were some videos he had uploaded to Pornhub. Alas, the plot thickens ... In the end, not wanting to risk Mr. Penis infecting me with spyware, malware, or some other form of cyber syphilis, I deleted all the emails he sent me.

---

[2] Jing Wu, Simin Li, and Hongzhe Wang. From Fans to "Little Pink" in Hailong Liu ed. *From Cyber-Nationalism to Fandom Nationalism: The Case of Diba Expedition in China.* New York: Routledge, 2020. Pg. 32.

[3] https://www.youtube.com/watch?v=0EGOJFQpfrs&t=57s

On Twitter an account appeared in April called "Fangfang Wuhandiary" (@wuhandiary), with a description "The Author of Wuhan Diary" and a photo of Fang Fang. I immediately texted Fang Fang to see if the account was legitimate; she responded by telling me that not only did she not have a Twitter account, but she didn't even know how to use a VPN to access Twitter! Then a second "Fang Fang" appeared on Twitter, this one with the handle "Fangfang_wuhandiary" (@fangfang_wuhan), and began reporting news from official state-run media sources like China Xinhua News and CGTN and posting propagandistic counter-messages, like:

Could the US please just carry on their election not mentioning China? Could they just mind their own business? Could the UK leave hk alone and mind their own matters? (4/25/20)

America has So many reporters and CIA agents in China (don't deny it, I know you do). They don't give you information? When you start to make decisions by the information Chinese government gave you? I didn't know your government trust Chinese government that much. (5/2/20)

I just had a phone call with a friend in new York, he told me that he is so terrified now. there are trucks carrying dead bodies everywhere. You can even feel the smell sometimes. People suddenly pass away while walking on the street. OMG. (5/3/20)

if Chinese government want to hide something, do you even think the wuhan diary (which I have to make clear is not true) full of dark side of the story could get published, and the author living in China with great wealth provided by the government (which I cannot imagine as well). (5/4/20)

So now there were fake Fang Fangs on Twitter spewing propaganda, even claiming, in the author's name, that "her" own book was "not true."

I began to see a huge uptick in unsolicited emails and texts from Chinese writers looking for an English translator. There is nothing inherently out of the ordinary about that; every year I tend to receive several such messages but now there was an explosion. And because of all the incessant attacks on the book, many authors who clearly self-identified as "anti-China" started to write to me. Most of those inquiries made me feel just as uncomfortable as the trolls. I would begin to feel uneasy when I received emails and private messages like: "…my novel is about freedom, democracy, and the struggle for human rights and universal fraternity; it is a revolt against dictatorship and hegemony. I'm sure it will win the adoration of the people of the world." Is this another Alex Penis trolling me? Was I growing paranoid? This also speaks to an ancillary side effect of mass online trolling campaigns, that is, the act itself undermines other forms of online communication and exchange.

Meanwhile, the trolls on Chinese social media were working overtime, claiming I had a history of posting "anti-China" comments on Twitter and Facebook. References to fictional Twitter posts that I never wrote were attributed to me and widely circulated online. One attack post even dug through my Facebook newsfeed, took multiple screenshots, and uploaded the content to Weibo with a narrative thread aimed at providing "evidence" of my anti-China tendencies. One of the posts cited as "evidence" was an article from CNN about changing conceptions of masculinity in China, which I had shared on my Facebook wall with no commentary. Was reposting an article about gender in China the smoking gun that I was part of the new "anti-China clique"? Was this "evidence" of my anti-China bias? But it didn't matter, many Weibo users are unable to read the original content; it is the slanderous talking points touted by the trolls that stick. Alas, I had become a target of "human-flesh search." Besides the sense of violation that people were methodically combing through my past social media posts with the malicious intention of digging up potentially damaging information, the truly insidious part of these posts is the fact that most Chinese netizens have no access to Twitter and Facebook and therefore have absolutely no way of independently authenticating these stories, which are instead blindly accepted as truth by many internet users. Sadly for many Weibo users, seeing a slickly edited post with ample screenshots in a foreign language, framed by an aggressive Chinese narrative announcing my crimes, was ample "evidence."

As *Wuhan Diary* made headlines, I began to get invitations to deliver online lectures about my experience translating the book. And, for the first time in my career, I also began to get "uninvited" from events or asked to "revise my topic" as the book became increasingly controversial. Between April and June 2020, I was uninvited or asked to revise my topic on five separate occasions, including one university in the United States. The US university never provided a formal reason why the event was cancelled, but the organizer did mention concern from colleagues about how the lecture might negatively impact their satellite campus in China. The long shadow of fear and intimidation which had emanated from the witch hunt launched on Chinese social media was now manifested here at home. In the meantime, I continued to grant interviews and deliver talks when invited. After having witnessed the devastating impact of the long-running disinformation campaign, I was intent on speaking out whenever I had a platform to do so; but even then, things did not go quite as I had anticipated.

On July 2, 2020, Radio France Internationale (RFI) broadcast an extensive interview they had conducted with me in Chinese. The interview was an attempt to correct many of the lies and conspiracy theories surrounding *Wuhan Diary*. I uploaded a link to my Weibo account and within just four or five hours the post had been read 340,000 times … and then it was deleted. Once the actual interview, my words, my defense, were scrubbed from the internet, then came the attacks. Professor Zhang Yiwu, who had been posting about Fang Fang since March 2020, uploaded the first of several attacks against me on July 6. Throughout his long response to my interview, which ran nearly 2000 characters, he repeatedly attempted to reinforce his view that I was the one being deceitful and further pushed his conspiracy theories concerning the book. Zhang wrote: "…he openly deceives and twists facts on Chinese readers, taking those fierce attempts to blame China and extremely aggressive essays as actions of kindness towards China. In this sense this translator is just like Fang Fang; they are both openly lying and deceiving Chinese society." He then goes on to argue:

The translator has the nerve to attack critics of Fang Fang's diary by saying: 'They are all spreading rumors and the talking points of the ultra-leftists are all lies.' Actually, the only ones making up lies and fabricating stories are Fang Fang and her translator. What this translator wants to hide most is the lie that Fang Fang's diary has triggered strong dissatisfaction in the Chinese-speaking world, which is also the same fake news being widely spread in the West. In that world the sole source of information on that "pile of abandoned cellphones" is a lie; the blame she puts on numerous Wuhan doctors; and the way she spread news of nurse Liang Xiaoxia's 梁小霞 death without an ounce of proof. These are the central items that have led the Chinese-speaking world to have reservations about Fang Fang's diary, yet the translator dares not respond or face them. The bold lies that Fang Fang has wantonly spread have now been transmitted around the world by this translator who has no regard for the reservations the Chinese-speaking world has for them; the intention is clearly to attack Chinese society. He dares not face the true suspicions and instead just keeps repeating how people have called him names like "white pig" and "CIA agent." This translator is attempting to convince the world to believe that everyone criticizing Fang Fang's diary in China is an ultra-leftist or a nationalist. Actually, what he should do is ask

Fang Fang to show us that photograph of the "abandoned cellphones," which she can never do because then the underhanded lies that he and Fang Fang have attempted to pass off to the world would be revealed. He no longer has even the slightest amount of academic integrity left, just as Fang Fang has not even a shred of literary integrity left to her name.

I was immediately reminded of that article in *Service Report*, published more than 25 years earlier. Back then there was something innocent, almost cute, about that doctored report, but this time the malicious tone of Zhang Yiwu's post left me speechless. The seemingly fatal flaws of the diary (the cellphone photograph, blame on doctors, and news of Liang Xiaoxia's death) are all items Fang Fang has repeatedly addressed in her diary (and in later interviews). The cellphone photo was shared by a friend of hers and unless that individual decides to release it, she had no right to make the image public; the only doctors she blamed in her diary were hospital administrators who she believed should be investigated due to their early failure to protect their own staff and employees; and the issue of Liang Xiaoxia was a mistake, which Fang Fang apologized for in the pages of her diary. What is more interesting is the fact that Zhang Yiwu insists on perpetuating an absurdist logic where layer upon layer of lies is used to bury the truth. I also found it interesting how Zhang never once referred to me by name in his essay, instead repeatedly addressing me as "the translator." When in reality, he knows me; I even translated *his* essay!

It was 1996 and I was still an undergraduate when I first attempted a serious translation project. I was in my senior year at Rutgers University and my professor Xudong Zhang was guest editing an issue of the academic journal *Boundary 2*. He asked me if I might be willing to consider translating an article for the special issue. I hadn't given serious thought to translation before that point, but the prospect enticed me. Professor Zhang even had to get special permission for an undergraduate to contribute to the journal. The essay I ended up translating—it became my first published work—was "Postmodernism and Chinese Novels of the Nineties" by Peking University Professor Zhang Yiwu. Over the course of translating the essay, I encountered a bevy of new theoretical terms like "Post-New Era" (*Hou xinshiqi* 後新時期) and was introduced to a group of new generation Chinese writers. I was so excited and motivated that I not only translated his essay, but tracked down all of the novels and short stories he discussed in the essay and began voraciously reading the works of writers like Xu Kun 徐坤, Han Dong 韓東, and Liu Xinglong 劉醒龍. I also bought a copy of Zhang Yiwu's own book *From Modernity to Postmodernity*

(*Cong xiandaixing dao houxiandaixing* 從現代性到後現代性). In some ways, it was through the experience of translating Zhang's essay that I began to cement my own future career trajectory as a scholar and translator. Not long after translating the essay, I actually met Zhang Yiwu when he visited Rutgers for a lecture. We had a nice conversation and he affectionately referred to me as "Xiao Bai 小白," a nickname that many of my friends and professors called me back then. I had long fallen out of touch with Professor Zhang Yiwu, although I did reach out to him on Weibo a few years ago and we had a cordial exchange. I was aware that in recent years, Zhang Yiwu had reinvented himself as an influential public intellectual, hosting television shows, earning an army of followers on Chinese social media, and aligning himself with an increasingly leftist political agenda. But even more than two decades later, I always had a soft spot for Zhang Yiwu because my career as a translator had begun with his work. I'm not sure if I would have ever had the confidence to tackle Yu Hua's *To Live* (*Huozhe* 活著)—the first novel I translated, which I began as a college senior—had it not been for that earlier experience translating Zhang Yiwu's essay. So you can guess my surprise when his name started appearing in Fang Fang's diary as one of the more high-profile voices attacking her; even more surprising was when he came after me.

I hope he knows that the passion, dedication, and attention to detail that I brought to *Wuhan Diary* is the exact same commitment I brought to his essay more than 20 years earlier. Surely Zhang must understand that the translation of a historical document (which is how I viewed Fang Fang's account) does not necessarily constitute an ideological endorsement of all content contained within. But it is difficult to have a civilized debate with an ideologue intent on carrying out personal attacks and character assassination.

It is worth noting that although Zhang Yiwu was posting his attacks from his personal Weibo account, besides his title as Professor of Chinese Literature at Peking University, he also holds a number of influential political posts; Zhang is a member of the 13th National Committee of Culture, History, and Learning; a representative of the 15th Beijing Municipal People's Congress; Deputy Director of the Committee of Education, Science, Culture, Health and Sports; member of the Central Committee of Democratic Progressives; Deputy of the Committee of Culture and Art; Deputy Chairman of the Beijing Municipal Committee for China's Democratic Progress; and the list goes on. Given the number of high-level titles Zhang holds, it is difficult to fathom someone like him spending so much time attacking a diary, unless of course, it was somehow part of his political mission.

But Zhang wasn't done yet. His attacks against me would intermittently continue over the course of the next couple of months, and on September 14, 2020, hours after I delivered an online lecture at "COVID-19 and Beyond, Culturally Speaking," an international conference hosted by Hong Kong Baptist University, Zhang was at it again. He uploaded a scathing essay, complete with screenshots of my talk, where the core ideas of my lecture were completely distorted and twisted. Instead, Zhang characterized my talk, which was an attempt to analyze the controversy surrounding *Wuhan Diary* in the following way:

> At this important event the most eye-catching presentation was from the first speaker, which was the translator of Fang Fang's diary, Michael Berry. He was yet again enthusiastically promoting Fang Fang's diary in a manner completely outside the framework of normal academic discussion; instead he viciously attacked Wuhan and China. Moreover, he slandered and cursed the criticisms that China and the Chinese people from all over the world have waged against the book's lies; he is an aggressor just like Pompeo and his talk was completely devoid of any academic discussion.[4]

And that was just the beginning. Throughout his 1500-word essay, Zhang proceeded to create his own fabricated narrative around my slides. For instance, in my lecture I explained how although topics like "the origin of the virus" and "Sino-US tensions" were *not* discussed by Fang Fang at all in her diary, they had become central talking points for the trolls, who had artificially pulled the diary into those debates. However, in Zhang's summary it becomes: "He raised the very important question of who gets to control the narrative of the Wuhan outbreak; from his perspective Fang Fang is the *only* authentic voice. He also mentioned the current tension in Sino-US relations, the controversy over the origin of the virus, and debates about civil society within Chinese society, etc. It is against this framework that he feels Fang Fang's diary has importance global significance."[5] This is Zhang's basic strategy, borrowing keywords, phrases, and ideas from my talk, but then restructuring them to fit into an argument completely antithetical to my original points. His rhetoric builds throughout the essay culminating in more comparisons to Mike Pompeo and the proclamation that "this person's words are brimming with animosity toward Chinese society, lacking in even a tiny sliver of academic analysis, and instead uses

---

[4] https://www.weibo.com/1194868525/JkRmC550N?type=comment#_rnd16028 23598082
[5] Ibid.

Fang Fang's diary as a tool to promote propaganda in an academic environment."⁶ In the face of these attacks, part of me could not help but feel a sense of sadness. Zhang Yiwu was a scholar that, once upon a time, at the very beginning of my academic career, I had greatly respected and admired. Now, more than two decades later, here he was spreading vile and vicious lies and rumors about me. Over time, I was also struck by a sense of pity. Here was a man so consumed by pure ideology; everything he perceived was in black or white, and there was absolutely no recognition of the violence he was unleashing with each and every post. As an "academic influencer" with more than nine million followers on Weibo, his every post would trigger another wave of attacks and often death threats targeting me and my family in the form of private messages. As he repeatedly depicted me as a hate-filled ideologue, spreading rumors, seeding lies, promoting conspiracy theories, and utterly devoid of academic integrity, it increasingly became clear that he was talking about himself. But there was no doubt that the deeper I got pulled into this cycle of meta-attacks, the more absurd the whole affair became. They manufacture lies, I attempt to correct the lies with accurate information and context, which is in turn labeled as "fake news," and so the cycle continues.

It is also worth stepping back to reflect upon the forces that have led Chinese intellectuals like Zhang Yiwu to take this "leftist" turn. Throughout the 1980s and into the 1990s, the cultural landscape in China was extremely diverse. It was common to see liberal-leaning works of cultural criticism like *The Silent Majority* (*Chenmo de dadoushu* 沉默的大都数) by Wang Xiaobo 王小波 in bookstores alongside hawkish titles like *China Can Say No* (*Zhongguo keyi shuobu* 中国可以说不). But since the Xi Jinping era, space for cultural discourse has retracted, with more stringent censorship, tighter control of the media and the internet, and "greater rewards" for those intellectuals who "play by the rules." It is not a simple case of repression, but a more complex result of the interplay between the carrot and the stick—artists, intellectuals, and activists are left to choose between pushing the boundaries and risk losing their platform, their voice, their livelihood, or aligning their values, discourse, and activities with those of the state and be rewarded. As China's post-2000 economic rise has gained momentum, the incentives for intellectuals who play by the rules have increased: a celebrity public intellectual who actively promotes the "positive energy" platform can host television shows and podcasts, endorse products, go on large-scale lecture tours, be appointed to high-ranking political positions, etc. The rebels are rewarded

⁶ Ibid.

with obscurity. This dynamic has been further accelerated under Xi Jinping. It has also, to some extent, been institutionalized: in 2019 Peking University, where Zhang Yiwu teaches, actually amended their charter to replace references to "academic freedom" with "a pledge of loyalty to the…Chinese Communist Party."[7] In 2020 similar changes were instituted at universities throughout China. Thus this leftist turn in Chinese academia is increasingly becoming not just encouraged, but incumbent. Further accentuating this trend is the exile or self-exile of numerous liberal-leaning cultural figures who had played a key role as public intellectuals from the 1980s to the 2000s, but whose influence was marginalized if not erased within China after going abroad.[8] It is against this backdrop that an increasing number of Chinese intellectuals have made the calculated decision to prioritize "political correctness" over objective research, "positive energy" over critical discourse, and "wolf warrior" discourse over civil engagement.

Eventually, the cycle of attacks started to gradually shift. Any and all book reviews and articles about *Wuhan Diary* started to generate personal attacks aimed at me. When Peter Hessler published a *New Yorker* article (unrelated to Fang Fang) entitled "How China Controlled the Coronavirus" on August 17, 2020, trolls lauded him by saying how much better his account was than "that stupid cunt Michael Berry"; but two months later, when Hessler published a second *New Yorker* article, "Nine Days in Wuhan, the Ground Zero of the Coronavirus Pandemic," in which he interviewed Fang Fang and discussed *Wuhan Diary*, the trolls immediately changed their tenor with posts like "no matter how many writers like Michael Berry and Peter Hessler that the American fascists hire, their words will never be able to bring back the 210,000 lives that have been lost." Attacks also became even more unbridled and removed from any sense of reality: When Ian Johnson published "China's bureaucracy controlled the pandemic. But some see Chinese flaws in the authoritarian state" in *The New York Review of Books*, Zhang Yiwu wrote: "Fang Fang, this person lacking in even the most basic human dignity, has here in this essay made her intentions to serve as an underhanded tool for the West to attack China as clear as can be."

[7] Gao Feng and Wong Lok-to. "Top Chinese Universities Amend Charters to Remove Reference to Freedom" *Radio Free Asia*. December 18, 2019. https://www.rfa.org/english/news/china/academic-freedom-12182019141313.html

[8] A partial list of prominent Chinese cultural figures who have left China includes Ai Weiwei 艾未未, Cui Zi'en 崔子恩, Liao Yiwu 廖亦武, Liu Binyan 劉賓雁, Liu Zaifu 劉再復, Wang Ruowang 王若望, Zhu Rikun 朱日坤, etc.

Later, the range of attacks would expand so that all kinds of negative news from the United States would become a platform to attack me, such as when *New Yorker* writer and CNN legal analyst Jeffrey Toobin was embroiled in a 2020 scandal after allegedly masturbating during a Zoom meeting, Weibo trolls posted a purported screenshot images of his genitals (likely not from the actual Toobin call) with a message to me "Is that what all you Americans do?" Or during the height of Russian-Ukraine War in 2022 when Russian media claimed the United States sponsored biolabs in Ukraine (dismissed by most Western media outlets as disinformation), trolls demanded that I "explain America's stance on using bioweapons!!!". The vast majority of these critical posts had absolutely no connection to *Wuhan Diary*; instead, my Weibo message thread and private message box seemed to transform into a clearinghouse for any and all anti-American content. These included a November 18, 2020, article on Weibo posted by Observer Network about Texas prison inmates being used to transport the bodies of COVID-19 victims with the comment "Democracy is dead. Who will liberate the suffering Americans?" in which both Fang Fang and I were tagged. Even when the bulk of attacks died down, a few straggler trolls using anonymous names like "Flight News (本航新聞)," "Feifan Wedding Photography (feifan 婚禮攝影)," and "German Farmer (德國農夫)" continued to tag me in critical posts and comments on an almost daily basis well into 2022. In January 2021, as the one-year anniversary of the Wuhan lockdown approached, various Western media outlets published a series of "one year later" themed reports; the WHO also sent an investigative team to Wuhan to investigate the source of the initial outbreak; all of this further inflamed attacks against *Wuhan Diary*. As more time passed since the original appearance of the diary and with online discourse concerning *Wuhan Diary* inundated with nearly a year of critical articles, the attacks became increasingly audacious and removed from reality. Allegations against the book began to expand from simple claims that Fang Fang's account was slanderous or based on hearsay to bolder claims that she was trying to use her diary to undermine the legitimacy of the Chinese Communist Party or incite a "colour revolution" in China!

One of Fang Fang's most vocal critics, Sima Nan, a popular television personality and political pundit, released a vlog on January 28, 2021, attacking the author. In describing those who supported Fang Fang and her novel *Soft Burial*, Sima Nan claimed: "what they are doing is not exercising some abstract notion aimed at protecting freedom of expression; they are trying to negate the Chinese revolution! They are trying to exercise their freedom to negate the very legal foundation of the People's Republic of China!" Or when quoting a Chinese literary prize jury that lauded *Soft Burial*'s "critical spirit," Sima Nan rhetorically asked: "So just what is this novel criticizing? It is criticizing the very political foundation of the People's Republic of China!"[9] Such incendiary claims repeatedly painted Fang Fang as a "counter-revolutionary" or a "traitor to China," all labels that harken back to the Mao era and the Cultural Revolution. Sima Nan makes all of this clear in the conclusion to the same vlog where he put out an open invitation for Fang Fang to appear on his program to explain:

> ...how she has gone against the revolution, how she has gone against the Chinese Land Reform Movement, and how she has challenged the very political foundation of the People's Republic of China. In order to win international awards, she has led her country to repeatedly suffer; in order to lend credence to those international voices intent on vilifying China, you keep handing them knives to hurt us! As I come to the end of my program, I must say: Fang Fang, you are wrong! You should reflect upon what you have done! If that day of reflection is not today, perhaps tomorrow that turning point will come. And if it doesn't, as Chairman Mao said: 'Some people are intent upon bring their stubbornness to the grave.'[10]

These comments, released a full year after the first installment of *Wuhan Diary*, were uploaded to Weibo to show not only the protracted nature of the attacks, but also how, over time, the crimes against Fang Fang had evolved. Not only were Sima Nan's broad and baseless claims far detached from anything in her published writings but they also allege that Fang Fang was inciting subversion of state power, a serious charge that has resulted in jail sentences for many dissidents in China. Sima's attacks also display a distinctly performative side: besides his activities in politics, Sima Nan is actually a television and film actor. (His real name is Yu Li 于力 and Sima Nan is his stage name.) His political videos also embellish his acting skills as he frequently shows off different accents to mock the targets of his attacks, which he punctuates with condescending smirks and laughter reminiscent of Nan Batian 南霸天 and other villains from socialist era cinema. One year after the initial release of *Wuhan Diary*, Sima Nan claimed that "not only has Fang Fang handed the knife over the West, but now she

[9] Sima Nan: Critique of Fang Fang Being Awarded the Emile Guimet Prize for Asian Literature (Sima Nan: Ping Fang Fang you huo Faguo Jimei wenxuejiang) January 28, 2021. https://www.youtube.com/watch?v=dnrqtRXTPRg
[10] Ibid.

herself has *become* the knife to impale China!"[11] But Sima Nan was not alone: other attacks appearing during the one-year anniversary of the Wuhan lockdown went even further.

As the online chatter and political rhetoric against Fang Fang escalated, articles and posts also began to shift from empty allegations to concrete calls for government action to be taken against Fang Fang. In a series of viral online articles, Wang Cheng 王誠 wrote, "Fang Fang may be a dog in the water, but isn't dead yet. We should keep in mind what Lu Xun said about mercilessly beating those dogs in the water! Otherwise they could bite you as soon as they get back on shore! So let's all work together to beat down that dog in the water! [...] I strongly suggest that the investigative branch of the public security bureau, acting in accordance of relevant legal codes, investigate Fang Fang for the crime of attempting to overturn state power and figure out the exact extent to which she colluded with external forces...."[12] Zhang Hongliang 張宏良, a professor at Minzu University of China, called for similar steps to be taken when he wrote:

Fang Fang is an anti-communist class enemy, she is an anti-China traitor to the nation; there is no question about this. The main question right now is: who allowed this anti-communist and anti-China element to ever assume the rank of a provincial-level cadre? What were the factors that allowed her anti-communist publications to actually win literary awards? And who gave her the power to operate outside the confines of the law? According to the legal code, those who spread rumors during a time of a pandemic outbreak are to be sentenced to seven years in prison. And during the entire period of the pandemic there was no greater rumor-monger than Fang Fang....[13]

Quoting a series of blogs and Weibo posts, the vlogger who goes by the name Xingzai shuo Zhongguo 幸仔說中國, or "Lucky Talks China," posted a viral video with even more outrageous claims:

One member of the American media has begun to attack Fang Fang! He claims that Fang Fang has misled the United States, leading the Americans to believe that COVID-19 was the result of human error. This caused the United States to not take the virus seriously, ultimately resulting in the cataclysmic

---

[11] Ibid.

[12] Feng Yunkan. "Check Out Which Specialists Support Fang Fang and Who is Against Her" ("Kankan zhichi he fandui Fang Fang de zhuanjia dou you shei?" 看看支持和反對方方的專家都有誰?) https://zhuanlan.zhihu.com/p/133760882

[13] Ibid.

spread of COVID-19. I suspect that in the not too distant future we will be seeing lawsuits brought against Fang Fang on behalf of the United States!... Fang Fang has played a role in setting the entire world off on the wrong direction [regarding COVID-19] and enabling Western society to numb themselves to the differences between themselves and their understanding of China....[14]

Alas, the ultimate destination of a year of twisted and slanderous lies against Fang Fang culminated in accusations that she not only transformed herself into an ideological and political weapon to harm China, but that she was to blame for the United States' (and the entire Western world's) failure to control COVID-19! Such has been the arc of the political attacks against Fang Fang.

"Lucky Talks China" posted another viral video on January 23, 2021, where he actually created a fictionalized narrative about how Trump had been hoodwinked by *Wuhan Diary*, directly contributing to the United States' failure to control the outbreak! As Lucky recounted in his video:

At 9:00am on April 17, 2020, Trump strolled into his White House office right on time and, before he could even sit down behind the resolute desk, he picked up the phone and called the head of the FBI. The moment the call went through, Trump's face turned red with anger as he yelled into the phone: "You worthless idiots! What kind of shitty intelligence reports have you been providing me with? Just yesterday I announced that we must all get back to work on May 1!" With that, Trump opened up his desk drawer and removed the top secret file that the FBI had sent him: *Fang Fang's Diary*. "Don't tell me we have been duped by Fang Fang's diary?" Trump slipped into a period of deep thought.[15]

---

[14] This quotation and the allegations contained within were originally posted on the Chinese social media platform Weibo but later quoted and amplified through viral vlog posts uploaded to YouTube and other streaming sites. It was quoted at length in the video post "After a Full Year of Making a Scene, When Will Fang Fang Get What is Coming to Her? Today We Have an Answer!" ("Fang Fang naoteng le yi nian, shenme shihou shoushi ta? Jintian you daan!" 方方鬧騰了一年，什麼時候收拾她?今天有答案!) by Xingzai Shuo Zhongguo 幸仔說中國 (Lucky Talks China) on February 2, 2021. https://www.youtube.com/watch?v=iI4NBPWR95g.

[15] See Xingzai shuo Zhongguo's 幸仔說中國 (Lucky Talks China) vlog "Three Days After Biden Assumes Office, the United States has Suddenly Realized there is a Serious Problem! Fang Fang has Terribly Deceived them! Life in China is Good!" ("Baideng shangtai 3 tian, Meiguo turan yishidao yige zhongyao wenti! Fang Fang ba tamen piancan le! Shenghuo zai Zhongguo zhen xingfu!" 拜登上台3天，美國突然意識到一個重要問題!方方把他們騙慘了!生活在中國真幸福!) January 23, 2021 on YouTube: https://www.youtube.com/watch?v=6Mjljle795Q.

Lucky's account, uploaded on exactly the one-year anniversary of the Wuhan lockdown, came amid this new wave of online strikes. It also represented a new level of even more unbridled attacks on Fang Fang and a new level of conspiracy theories, even more divorced from reality which went so far as blaming the Western world's failure in controlling on COVID-19 outbreak on Fang Fang.

It might be tempting to write these fanciful attacks off as so removed from reality that no even-minded reader could ever entertain as truth; however, these conspiratorial fabrications have a tendency to grow, spread, and morph over time, often borrowing kernels of truth to make them seem more authentic.[16] Six months after Lucky Talks China first began to promote the idea that Fang Fang had somehow fallen out of favor with the United States and was being blamed for COVID-19 deaths in the United States, the story took yet another twist. On July 26, 2021, the Chinese military blogger Yizhiliulian 一纸琉涟 posted the following Weibo essay, which immediately went viral:

> U.S. Congressman Davis requested that Congress implement sanctions, order the arrest, and detention of the Chinese writer Fang Fang, claiming that it was Fang Fang's erroneous views that misled the United States, leading to more than 34 million official cases of COVID-19 in the United States and causing more than 610,000 deaths. Davis pointed out that Fang Fang deliberately spread misinformation about the uselessness of masks, the uselessness of city-wide lockdowns, and the uselessness of quarantine measures during the early stages of the COVID-19 epidemic; she instead made false claims such as freedom and democracy were the best means to fight the epidemic. Davis pointed out that the United States has suffered the more from COVID-19 than any other country in the world and has the worst response record when it comes to preventive measures. This is primarily due to being misled by Fang Fang'. Therefore, he called upon the White House to bring Fang Fang to justice as soon as possible by extraditing Fang Fang to the United States for trial.
>
> The views of the American congressmen are indeed quite peculiar. The United States and Britain gave Fang Fang a very high evaluation at the

---

[16] A good example of using a kernel of truth to make exaggerated claims can be seen in the repeated allegations made by hundreds of trolls online that I was "paid off" or "rewarded" with an $80,000 payment by the US government for translating Fang Fang's diary. In reality, months before Fang Fang began writing *Wuhan Diary*, I had applied to the National Endowment for the Arts for a Translation Grant to translate Fang Fang's novel *Soft Burial*. The grant application was selected for funding by an external jury made up of professional translators later in 2020. The amount of funding granted was $12,500 USD, roughly 80,000 yuan.

beginning, but now they blame Fang Fang for misleading the United States. The United States indeed has the worst record in terms of their response to the epidemic. The United States is also the country with the largest number of confirmed cases and deaths. What's more serious is that the US epidemic has caused a full-scale internal crisis in the United States, and the various fissures that have opened have reached the point where they can no longer be bridged. Due to the impact of the epidemic, the latest polls in the United States show that 55% of respondents believe that the future of the United States is bleak, and only 45% believe that the future is promising. More and more Americans have seen through the political propaganda to see Biden administration for what it is; the consensus is that Biden is incapable of solving the myriad problems that plague the United States.

Americans are becoming more and more pessimistic. This is caused by the United States' own extreme irresponsibility and the inevitable result of the arrogance of American politicians. Under these circumstances, there is no longer any reason for them to protect Fang Fang any longer; however it does seem a bit preposterous that an American congressman would decide to use Fang Fang as a scapegoat at a time like this. Of course, the fact that a U.S. congressman would accuse Fang Fang of these crimes and call for her arrest is a result that no one could have anticipated. Fang Fang has won the support of many individuals in the West, and the United States has also actively promoted Fang Fang. It is therefore indeed a surprise to see these sudden accusations being directed at Fang Fang by an American congressman.[17]

While echoing claims that had already been circulating six months earlier, this time the accusations were further "backed up" by a barrage of similarly fabricated articles, such as "Kill Her Off Now That the Job is Done! US Congressman Recommends Prosecuting Fang Fang; She Should Pay For the COVID-19 Outbreak in the US" (却磨杀驴!美国议员建议起诉方方，为美国疫情暴发买单),[18] a series of YouTube-style videos,[19] and widespread social media activity, which not only took the views espoused in these articles at face value, but widely endorsed and disseminated them. The message

---

[17] https://weibo.com/u/6284509007?topnav=1&wvr=6&topsug=1&is_hot=1#162743 0819742

[18] "Kill Her Off Now That the Job is Done! US Congressman Recommends Prosecuting Fang Fang; She Should Pay For the COVID-19 Outbreak in the US" (Quemo shalu! Meiguo yiyuan jianyi qisu Fang Fang, wei Meiguo yiqingbaofa maidan却磨杀驴!美国议员建议起诉方方，为美国疫情暴发买单) Published on Jianwen zixun 见闻资讯 on July 27, 2021. https://www.163.com/dy/article/GFUAA9UT0552CFHJ.html?f=post2020_dy_recommends

[19] Such as Haiqing's video commentary, which was uploaded to YouTube on July 27, 2021. https://www.youtube.com/watch?v=SwFD1AbxvUs

board on the Yizhiliulian's post includes thousands of comments like "It's fucking hilarious they paid her to dig a hole and now they've fallen into it," "They paid someone to do a job, she screwed it up and now they are killing her to shut her up and destroy the evidence!", and "Kill the dog now that it has outlived its usefulness!"—all of which speaks to the ability of these fabrications to be accepted as fact by many netizens.

While Chinese leftist detractors attempted to link stories like these to the *Wuhan Diary* controversy, such posts actually speak to much broader debates about government and society. In particular, posts about the failure of Western governments (particularly the United States) to control the COVID-19 outbreak, let alone even offer a unified federal response, were repeatedly framed in the larger context of the failure of the Western democratic model. Juxtaposed against China's aggressive response and successful control of COVID-19, such posts emphasize the final triumph of "socialism with Chinese characteristics," "proving" it to be a more effective political model than liberal Western democracies and strengthening the legitimacy of a political system that has often been maligned and attacked in the West as authoritarian, autocratic, lacking transparency, and un-democratic. After decades of navigating controversial internal and external debates about political reform, it would take a global pandemic to unleash what, for many Chinese citizens, would be the most potent and irrefutable vindication of the Chinese political system's primacy over that of the Western democratic superpowers. After many critics had initially pointed to the Wuhan outbreak as a possible "Chernobyl moment" for the Chinese Communist Party, the abysmal failure of Western countries to contain COVID-19 in 2020 not only turned that narrative around, but it had opened up an opportunity for the CCP to double down and offer a sweeping censure on the shortcomings of democracy itself as a political system. In other words, the controversies surrounding COVID-19 became a de facto public referendum on different forms of political systems, ultimately further tightening Xi Jinping's grip on power and reinforcing the Chinese public's support of the party, even as the CCP navigated controversial waters in Xinjiang and Tibet. (Two years later, much of the political capital earned early on would be compromised by a series of harsh lockdowns in Shanghai and other cities).

One of the strangest occurrences came when I started to appear as a character in Yam Bear Six's "American Diary." Installment 98 of "American Diary" was entitled "Square Not Round's Western Translator Has Betrayed Square Not Round"; "Square Not Round" (Fang bu yuan 方不圓) was a satirical reference to Fang Fang, which literally can mean "square" in Chinese, and I of course was the "Western translator." After another typical diary entry containing various revelations about Donald Trump's failures, Yam Bear Six concluded his entry with a commentary on my interview with Radio France Internationale, which had aired the previous day. Yam Bear catalogued what he deemed to be three jaw-dropping revelations from my interview—a translation of *Soft Burial* was in progress, Fang Fang indeed planned to donate her profits from the diary to charity, and the English version of the diary would not include her essay series "About" ("Guanyu")— (oh, the scandal of it all!) before ending with the following:

> In conclusion, there is something I want to raise a question about: Square Not Round's Western Translator Michael Berry stated that he wants to be a bridge between Chinese and Western culture; he wants to help China and Wuhan. We here in China have an old saying, "courtesy demands reciprocity!" Now that you in America have 2.8 million confirmed cases of COVID-19 and 130,000 deaths, I would also like to help you Americans, I would like to help New York. I wonder if this Western Translator will help me translate my "American Diary?" I feel my "American Diary" will be of much more help to America than Square Not Round's *Wuhan Diary* will ever be!!![20]

Courtesy indeed demands reciprocity and I humbly offer a translated excerpt of American Diary above. I would also be remiss not to also talk about the United States, which I address later in this book. Over the ensuing months, Yam Bear Six and his followers would continue to taunt me online, alternately asking me to translate his blog or to write my own "American Diary." In response to a Voice of America interview with me published on January 22, 2021, Yam Bear would devote an entire installment of his diary to attacking me. The entry, episode 298, entitled "Michael Berry, Why don't you be America's Fang Fang?" concluded with the following:

> Finally, I want to say: Michael Berry said that a strong country should be tolerant! But I want to say that China has tolerated Fang Fang, but America has not tolerated Donald Trump – they even banned him on Twitter! Fang Fang has not tolerated the Chinese people; she curses them as ultra-leftists! And Michael Berry has not tolerated the Chinese people, he curses them as Little Pinks and members of the 50 Cent Army! Michael Berry has said that what Fang Fang did was quite rare and no matter what sacrifice, she insisted on pushing forward! What I want to say is that many average people have suffered terrible economic hardships and yet Fang Fang has made money by selling her book to the Eight Nation Alliance; what has she sacrificed?

[20] https://www.weibo.com/ttarticle/p/show?id=2309404522745898598449

Michael Berry, you compliment Fang Fang with such beautiful words; why don't you be America's Fang Fang? Or are you afraid that you will end up the victim of a mysterious "suicide" in the United States?[21]

Yam Bear Six's followers responded by inundating my Weibo feed with yet another wave of attacks. I was surprised by just how prominently the very act of translation was featured in their posts:

When will you write your American Diary? I'll translate it into Chinese for you at no charge! (January 27, 2021)

Professor Berry, when can we expect your USA Diary? Thank you for caring so much about the COVID-19 situation in China, but we here in China are doing just fine. Perhaps you should pay more attention to what is happening in the United States: you treat black lives like they don't matter and you practice genocide against American Indians, but you always protect White lives, don't you? (January 27, 2021)

Help me translate my American Diary; don't look down upon me with your mongrel eyes, or do you only translate for big shots like Fang Fang who live in private villas? (January 27, 2021)

Michael Berry, fuck your mother; Fang Fang may not understand English; but don't tell me you don't fucking understand Chinese? You wrote directly on the cover of the book that Wuhan was the origin of the virus! What is your ulterior motive behind brazenly lying with your eyes open? Fang Fang, the witch of lies, said you are an international friend of China, but from where I sit you are nothing but a spy! Not knowing any foreign languages certainly hasn't stopped bad Fang Fang from seducing a bad foreigner who does know a foreign language! Fuck! If you have the balls, write a book called *400,000 American Dead Souls* and see if you can still breath that air of freedom and democracy! Fuck! (January 27, 2021)

Michael Berry, you fucking shameless follower of Fang Fang; you are like a beggar that relies on translating Chinese essays by national traitors to earn some leftover scraps of food. You are a fucking criminal and God shall abandon you! You who go by the surname of Berry, your final destination shall be hell! It will be in the eighteenth level of hell! *Please translate that!* (January 29, 2021)

---

[21] Yam Bear Six 地瓜熊老六. "American Diary 298: Michael Berry, Why don't you be America's Fang Fang?" ("Meiguo riji 298: Bai Ruiwen, Ni weishenme bu zuo meiguo de Fang Fang" 美國日記298: 白睿文, 你為什麼不做美國的方方) January 28, 2021 on Weibo: https://weibo.com/ttarticle/p/show?id=2309404598468143612129#_0

Yam Bear Six's attacks became so potent that, in late July of 2022, while serving on the jury of one of China's largest independent film festivals, I was suddenly removed from the jury two days before the opening ceremony. The reason? Festival organizers gave in to threats and pressure waged by internet trolls unleased by Yam Bear Six. Shortly after a press release went out announcing the makeup of the jury, the trolls leapt into action, making it clear that I was none other than the translator of the "diary of lies," alleging that I was a US government operative, and rhetorically asking festival organizers if they were running a film festival or a CIA training camp. Once my photo and name were purged from the festival's website, Yam Bear Six promptly celebrated the "good news" on Weibo. What does it mean when the act of translation—an act built on the spirit of shared understanding, communication, and cultural exchange—becomes contorted and contaminated to the point that it is viewed as act of political aggression? The translation and publication of *Wuhan Diary* is in no way, shape, or form an attempt to "blame China," hurt China, or deflect attention away from the United States' own abysmal mishandling of COVID-19. That was a time when Americans were also in desperate need of help; in need of accurate reporting, effective leadership, and voices like Fang Fang's to hold American political leaders accountable for egregious failures, but I will come back to that.

Meanwhile, the elements of the strange online persecution continued to sneak into real life; an October report that arrests had been made in Qingdao after someone had spread rumors inflating the official number of COVID-19 cases in the city was forwarded by anti-Fang Fang trolls demanding that she face similar consequences for spreading rumors about "the abandoned cellphones" (not that again!); after large numbers of trolls filed official complaints about Fang Fang's alleged "illegal villa," an official investigation was launched (which did not find any wrongdoing on Fang Fang's part); and ultra-nationalist online attacks continued. While the witch hunt against Fang Fang was broader, was more protracted, and had caught the international media's attention, it was but one of numerous online campaigns being carried out on the Chinese internet in 2020. As nationalist aggression grew unfettered, many individuals were viciously targeted: leading Chinese epidemiologist Zhang Wenhong 張文宏 was attacked by nationalist trolls as "worshipping everything foreign" after he recommended Chinese children should improve their nutrition by consuming more milk and sandwiches for breakfast (instead of rice porridge); Chinese poets like Bei Dao 北島, arguably the single most important poet

of the Reform Era, and Yu Xiuhua 余秀華, who has overcome the challenges of cerebral palsy to win critical acclaim and several awards, were
both targeted online; *New Yorker* staff writer Jiayang Fan 樊嘉揚 wrote
about her own protracted struggle with Chinese trolls in the piece
"Motherland"; Hong Kong Baptist University Professor Tammy Lai-
Ming Ho 何麗明 was attacked for months because of her writings and
speech; and Tzu-I Chuang Mullinax 莊祖宜, a popular food blogger,
author of *The Anthropologist in the Kitchen* (*Chufang li de renlei xuejia* 廚
房裡的人類學家), and wife of the former US Consul General in Chengdu,
was attacked after some of her online essays were deemed "politically
incorrect." A round of attacks against the poet Jia Qianqian was launched
by Sima Nan and other trolls who had been targeting Fang Fang. And in
March 2021, after being widely lauded in China for her Academy Award
nomination, Chloe Zhao 趙婷 came under brutal attack by an army of
trolls that had dug up a few sentences from an old interview that they had
deemed "unpatriotic." When I saw how Zhao had been transformed from
a national hero to being vilified as a sell-out overnight, I was struck by the
similarities with what Fang Fang had experienced a year earlier. And in
both cases the troll attacks actually culminated in works being banned. It
is not a coincidence that, with the exception of Zhang Wenhong and Bei
Dao, all of the other individuals listed here—Yu Xiuhua, Jiayang Fan,
Tammy Ho, Tzu-I Chuang Mullinax, Chloe Zhao—are women. Many of
the online attacks feature a strong misogynist bent and are frequently filled
with threats of sexual violence, which was certainly true of the attacks on
Fang Fang and her "circle of friends" like Professors Liang Yanping and
Wang Xiaoni. In some sense, the fact I was targeted is merely as an exten-
sion, or perhaps collateral damage, of the main attacks being waged on
Fang Fang.

CHAPTER 10

Reasons

Given the unprecedented nature of these cyber-attacks, which were simultaneously carried out on multiple levels, from pseudo-academic "critical studies" of *Wuhan Diary* to anti-Fang Fang diss songs, looming large are the questions: **who was behind these attacks and what was at stake?** They are simple questions with a complex answer. Some media outlets in the West have made blanket statements blaming "the Chinese government" on the attacks; Fang Fang, on the other hand, has consistently attributed the attacks to the group she has labeled as "ultra-leftists." The truth is somewhat more complicated and murky. As in the case of *Soft Burial*, in which a relatively small group of radical pro-CCP ultra-leftists were able to successfully leverage their attacks into eventually getting the book removed from bookstores, it seems like the attacks on *Wuhan Diary* also began with a relatively small group of critics who were actively targeting both the blog and its author. Of course, tracing the origins of an online cyber campaign is a bit like trying to uncover the origins of COVID-19; but by tracing the authors of early critical posts and platforms in which they appeared, one can find a direct link between the group who attacked *Soft Burial* and some of the early posts critical of *Wuhan Diary*. However, unlike *Soft Burial*, which, while an important literary controversy covered by international press outlets like *The New York Times*, the novel never evolved into the kind of story that would become headline news around the world. As the *Wuhan Diary* blog gained popularity, Fang

M. Berry, *Translation, Disinformation, and Wuhan Diary*,
https://doi.org/10.1007/978-3-031-16859-8_10

Fang's critics and detractors also were able to leverage that popularity. After all, like a virus, or perhaps a parasite, these online trolls need a host. As their host (Fang Fang) gained in strength and popularity, so too their viral posts began to spread.

As installments of Fang Fang's diary became some of the most shared and discussed posts on Chinese social media from late January to early April, increasingly larger groups of internet trolls came to add fuel to the fire, fabricating an ever-growing list of controversial topics and later feeding on the carnage left behind. Because the vast majority of internet attacks do not come from individuals with real names, but instead are generated by attack accounts created under various pseudonyms like "User dzbfjrmca4," "PurpleFeatherDaddy," "Fang Fang Goes to Jail 方方進監獄了," "CrazyFattyGalle," "America is a Complete Failure 美國徹底失敗吧," "Big White Kitty and Big White Rabbit," and "WitnesstoHistory2020 見證歷史2020," it can be difficult to pinpoint exactly who is behind these accounts. Most of these users tend to have relatively few followers (from a few dozen to a few hundred) and many of their posts are dominated by nationalist content. For instance, "WitnesstoHistory2020" has a Weibo feed dominated by nationalist poster images, slogans like "Never Forget National Shame (毋忘國恥)," anti-Trump posts, and nostalgic images of Mao Zedong. But one thing many of them have in common is that they are all followers of a core group of extremely popular verified user accounts associated with an ultra-nationalist political stance that have millions of follows. These include "political influencers" on social media like Zhang Yiwu from Peking University (more than nine million followers); Yam Bear Six (more than six million followers); political commentator, scholar, and actor Sima Nan (more than two million Weibo followers); Xiang Ligang from CCTIME.COM (more than one million followers); as well as organizations/groups like Diba Expedition (more than one million followers). These political influencers exhibit a strong degree of coordination, often quoting one another in their respective posts and videos, echoing identical political talking points, and also simultaneously going after the same targets.[1] The unified talking points that different trolls parrot and the ways in which attacks are often unleashed simultaneously (often a deluge of hundreds or even thousands of messages are posted within the span of a few hours, sometimes just a few minutes) certainly speak to high degree of

---

[1] For instance, attacks on writer Jia Qianqian were simultaneously launched by Sima Nan, Yam Bear Six, and other troll accounts on January 31, 2021.

coordination and some form of top-down dissemination; it often reads as if trolls are following a script or a directive when launching attacks.

While difficult to make blanket generalizations, many of these users fall into one of several categories, including "ultra-leftists," "ultra-nationalists," "Little Pinks," and the "50 Cent Army." While Zhang Yiwu and others frequently object to Fang Fang's characterization of them as "ultra-leftists," it is a term with origins during the Cultural Revolution used to characterize political extremists fueled by a dogmatic nationalistic agenda. Some of these individuals have experienced the Mao era firsthand, such as Zhang Yiwu or the retired general who attacked *Soft Burial* in 2017. As discussed earlier, their online rhetoric often uses Mao-era political language and attack tactics, including the employment of Cultural Revolution-style propaganda posters, denunciation posters, witch hunt-like intimidation campaigns, and even WeChat groups with names like Little Red Soldiers. Overlapping with these "ultra-leftists" are broader groups of "ultra-nationalists" and "Little Pinks." While many of the so-called ultra-leftists display an open nostalgia for the political tactics of the Cultural Revolution, the "Little Pinks" are a generation of online activists who grew up under the economic prosperity of the post-1990s; they were too young to experience the political turmoil of 1989, let alone the Mao era. While the term dates back to 2008, the "Little Pinks" rose to prominence after a 2016 scandal involving Chou Tzu-yu 周子瑜, a Taiwanese pop star who was flooded by attacks after waving a Taiwan flag on television. According to journalist Zhuang Pinghui writing in 2017:

> Contrary to perceptions that most online patriots are angry young men, the Little Pink are mainly female. Some 83 per cent of these keyboard warriors identify as female, according to a Weibo analytics tool developed by Peking University. Research published by the Chinese Academy of Social Sciences says the Little Pink are predominantly young women aged between 18 and 24.[2]

While it is difficult to say if Little Pinks in 2020 and 2021, during the Fang Fang Incident, were still dominated by female internet users, they tend to be web-savvy and often utilize VPNs to express nationalist sentiment and launch attacks on platforms outside of China, including banned social

[2]Zhuang Pinghui. "The rise of the Little Pink: China's angry young digital warriors" South China Morning Post. May 26, 2017. https://www.scmp.com/news/china/society/article/2095458/rise-little-pink-chinas-young-angry-digital-warriors

media platforms like Facebook and Twitter. Another key to understanding how Fang Fang's popularity fueled additional online attacks is not relegated simply to political capital and online nationalism, there is also a monetary incentive. When stories go viral, attracting massive numbers of eyeballs and garnering millions of clicks, as was the case with *Wuhan Diary*, that also provides an opportunity for the so-called 50 Cent Army to make a buck. To explain how the 50 Cent Army functions, I turn to Chinese internet scholar Guobin Yang:

> …a new mechanism of "Internet Commentators" (*wangluo pinglun yuan* 網絡評論員) was introduced in 2004 to guide and influence the production of online opinion. Hired as volunteers or paid staff, these Internet commentators directly intervene in online discussions by writing responses to posts or joining the debates. Their mission, however, is not to promote critical debate but rather to covertly guide the direction of the debate in accordance with the principles laid down by the propaganda departments of the party. The guidance is covert, because internet commentators do not sign into online forums as such. Rather, they sign in with anonymous user IDs, like any other Internet user. Because of the deceptive role these internet commentators play, they have already earned themselves a bad name. The story goes that the government authorities pay an Internet commentator 50 cents (in RMD) for each message he or she posts in an online forum. Internet commentators have thus come to be known derogatively as the "fifty-cent party" (*wu mao dang*).[3]

While it can be difficult, if not impossible, to unravel just which attacks are generated by bots, trolls, genuine "patriotic" internet users, or the 50 Cent Party, the monetary incentive for the latter group certainly plays an important role in exponentially increasing attacks on topics which generate more hits. More importantly, as Liz Carter has observed, "The 50-Cent Party complicates China's online landscape, because its existence throws shadows of suspicion and doubt onto all facets of online debate. The knowledge that some pro-government posts are insincere undermines the credibility of all pro-government rhetoric."[4] Even the widely employed nickname used to describe these trolls nakedly speaks to the monetized

[3] Guobin Yang. *The Power of the Internet in China: Citizen Activism Online.* New York, Columbia University Press, 2009. Pgs. 50–51.
[4] Carter, Liz. *Let 100 Voices Speak: How the Internet is Transforming China and Changing Everything.* New York: I.B. Tauris, 2015. Pg. 54.

value of these online attacks. In addition to the 50 Cent Army, there are of course more standard ways in which viral videos criticizing Fang Fang can be monetized through ad revenue.

While so many of the online attacks are dominated by passionate political speech, racist and misogynistic comments, and hateful threats, there is also a strong sense of what might be characterized as "play" behind many of these posts. Many attacks use language in creative, subversive, and humorous ways, widely employing jokes, mockery, puns, and satire. Trolls banter among themselves, trying to "one up" each other in offering even more over the top attacks, putting forward increasingly creative conspiracy theories, and "exposing" even more scandalous "crimes." This is by no means an attempt to play down the seriousness of the attacks and the damaging impact they have, but there is clearly a strong undercurrent of playfulness and performance running through these posts. Whether they be young ultra-nationalists, members of the 50 Cent Party, Little Pinks, or ultra-leftists, some involved in the campaign against Fang Fang seem to approach the attacks as a form of online entertainment, an activity akin to playing video games or killing time in an online chat room. Part of this observation is indebted to my own participation on the app Clubhouse where I heard several groups devoted to comedic mockery of *Global Times* editor Hu Xijin. While there was certainly a strong political subtext that users were engaging with, even more palpable was the sense of "play" that they were bringing to the conversation. A similar sentiment of play runs through many of the online anti-Fang Fang posts, especially those of Yam Bear Six's "American Diary." By incorporating this undercurrent of "performative play" into serious political attacks, trolls are also able to garner more readers and active users who post and criticize not just in the name of ideology, but also for the "entertainment value" that such posts provide. This playful side of the attacks can also be readily seen in the robust series of works about Fang Fang that appeared in the realm of popular culture. By commenting on active threads, posting their own jokes and commentaries, and other forms of online participation, netizens not only gain a sense of engagement, but also a feeling of pleasure. The groundwork of publicly denouncing targets (in this case, Fang Fang) also opens up a space for average netizens to engage in these kinds of attacks without any sense of moral culpability since their target has already been "proven" to be an enemy, traitor, spy, profiteer, or any of the other labels that Fang Fang (or other targets) has been given over the course of these campaigns. The attacks become a form of violence that is sanctioned if not encouraged and, in the case of the 50 Cent Army, even rewarded monetarily.

With attacks being waged from so many different directions by so many disparate and loosely identified groups, there has been a lot of speculation as to whether the campaign against Fang Fang represents a top-down or bottom-up effort. Bondes and Schucher have argued that "…the majority of Chinese 'online mass incidents' develop entirely without the orchestration or engagement of any organization."[5] In this case, however, I would suggest that what eventually evolved was a more complex symbiotic dynamic wherein non-official discourse (online troll attacks, rumors, and parodies of Fang Fang) fueled official denunciations (critical articles published by *Global Times*, the People's Liberation Army, etc.), which, in turn, inspired more non-official attacks. The true turning point occurred when news of the international release of the book made headlines in early April. This is when Fang Fang's diary account underwent a sudden and radical transformation in terms of how that news was reported, received, and, in my view, twisted. The speed at which this shift took place can be traced in the pages of the government tabloid newspaper the *Global Times*; on March 19 editor Hu Xijin published an article largely praising the diary, even calling for "the nation to accept the 'Fang Fangs of every era'"[6] yet just a few weeks later, on April 8, Hu published a rather scathing editorial attacking the diary. The attacks published in the pages of that publication would continue to escalate as observed by Manoj Kewalramani:

> The vitriol can be gauged from the fact that at one point, *Global Times* carried a story mentioning social media debates comparing Fang Fang to Qin Hui, a Song Dynasty politician who treachery has been immortalized at a temple in Hangzhou. The site is home to the tomb of Yue Fei, a patriotic general, whom Qin and his wife had killed. Their statues kneel today outside the tomb, with tradition calling on passersby to spit at them.[7]

[5] Maria Bondes and Gunter Schucher, "Derailed emotions: The transformation of claims and targets during the Wenzhou online incident" in Wenhong Chen (ed.) *The Internet, Social Networks and Civic Engagement in Chinese Societies.* Routledge, 2015. pg. 46.

[6] Hu Xijin 胡錫進. "Huxijin's Take on the "Fang Fang Diary" Phenomena" ("Hu Xijin ping 'Fang Fang riji' xianxiang" 胡錫進評方方日記現象) Global Times 環球時報, March 19, 2020. https://news.ifeng.com/c/7uyH0zY3rsm

[7] Kewalramani, Manoj. *Smokeless War: China's Quest for Geopolitical Dominance.* New Delhi: Bloomsbury India, 2021. Pg. 65.

Overnight, what had previously been regarded as a national story was now also being pulled into the already present tensions between China and the United States, tensions which had no bearing on the diary itself as a literary record. However, it was also at this crucial junction, as anti Fang Fang rhetoric reached new heights, the massive number of social media posts and official news reports denigrating the diary also began to have a real impact in turning the tide of public opinion. It was at this point that attacks on Fang Fang were no longer fringe actions taken up by radical online political groups, but also began to sway the views of average netizens. With the pro-Fang Fang voices being suppressed, constructing a new online narrative critical of the book quickly gained traction. As China Digital Times editor Eric Liu observed, "The primary force of these attacks was certainly average Chinese netizens, but that is because their hatred was successfully harnessed."[8] Whereas public reactions to the diary were initially positive and later somewhat mixed, by the middle of April 2020 it was clear that this hate campaign was being centrally coordinated, which can be demonstrated by (1) the suddenness with which the more violent attacks began; (2) the scripted talking points that various attacks repeated; (3) unified messaging across not only different social media platforms, but also academic platforms and pop culture mediums; and (4) the way in which sharp spikes in the attacks were closely tied to ongoing (yet unrelated political events) like the "Two Sessions" in May of 2020 and the WHO-led investigation into the origin of COVID-19 in January of 2021, both of which triggered a large spike in the online attacks against *Wuhan Diary*.

Part of what further exacerbated the attacks were the practical circumstances of the COVID-19 outbreak in China. Millions of citizens were locked down at home where they were left angry, frustrated, and unable to work; meanwhile *everyone* was online. People were looking for a scapegoat, someone to blame, a place to project their frustrations and release their pent up anger—ideal conditions for a troll culture to fester and spread. The international edition of the book was announced just as the Wuhan lockdown was lifted and foreign nations were beginning to adopt a more aggressive and accusatory stance toward China; the timing made *Wuhan Diary* the perfect target for nationalist attacks. The rhetoric against Fang Fang was so powerful that I even received an email from one of my UCLA students from China who wrote to me to express his concern:

[8] Interview with Eric Liu, May 11, 2021.

I saw an online article about Fangfang Wuhan Diary and surprisingly I saw you translated it. And I'm a little curious about why you did it (There have been some conspiracy theories, but I wish to hear your true thoughts). You must already have known that this work and Fangfang have really infuriated the Chinese people (I say people here because some Western media seem to love framing it as the "government"). In fact, many Chinese people supported Fangfang at first for her courage to speak up but turned against her later because she seemed to tailor to certain interest groups (e.g. she kept depicting dead hope when stuff was already getting much better) and also because lots of the stories she wrote simply weren't true. I guess there should be no problem if people read it as a fiction, but I doubt if the Western audience are not taking it as "suppressed truth of what a totalitarian government wants to hide." I haven't read any of your translations, but I'm wondering if you've put any disclaimers like "The stories may have fictionate content" or that many of the facts are yet to be corrected? (*sic.*)

A few months later another one of my UCLA students from China again questioned my motivations for translating *Wuhan Diary*. He began by explaining, "I haven't actually read the diary, but from what I have read online…" and he proceeded to parrot the talking points that had been circulating online on Chinese social media and in official news reports. There was something particularly heartbreaking about seeing my own students repeating the bullet points the online trolls and disinformation campaign had laid out. But their comments, and those of so many others, show not only how effective the propaganda campaign against Fang Fang was, but also how even non-activist citizens became so incensed after reading the inundation of false news accounts of Fang Fang's so-called infractions that they felt a need to speak out, thus further fueling the online attacks and rampant spread of misinformation. What this transition also reveals is how quickly radical, conspiracy theory-laden, political views held by a small group of extremists can, through a sophisticated process of amplification, reiteration, and dissemination over a variety of different traditional and social media platforms, become accepted as mainstream ideology.

And then there is the question of what was at stake? The optics of sending death threats to a professor for translating a book can't be good. So what was it about the book that led to the mass mobilization of thousands of internet trolls and the production of slanderous pseudo-academic anti-Fang Fang books, rap songs, cartoons, and thousands of essays and online posts aimed at discrediting *Wuhan Diary*? There were multiple factors at work that played out simultaneously, in real time, as the diary was being written and as the COVID-19 outbreak unfolded. It was this dynamic confluence of forces that created the conditions for what would evolve into the so called Fang Fang Incident. The first directive goes back to Xi Jinping's imperative to tell "the good China story." In this case, *Wuhan Diary* unwittingly stepped into an ideological battle over who gets to control the narrative about the coronavirus outbreak in Wuhan. Fang Fang's account walked a tightrope between expressing support of government policies while also calling out local leaders and infectious disease specialists for missteps early on. As Hongwei Bao has observed, in contrast to other diary accounts by Wuhan-based writers like Ai Xiaoming and Guo Jing, *Wuhan Diary* was "probably the 'safest' because Fang never labeled herself as an activist-feminist or otherwise."[9] Fang Fang was a writer from the state system who knew all too well where the political lines were laid, yet somehow even her "careful" account would eventually prove to deviate too much from the script of "the good China story," a deviation which became exponentially exacerbated with news of the book's imminent international publication. There may have been objections to Fang Fang's story being told within in China, but the mere prospect that hers would be the story told to the world was unacceptable.

There were several features that made Fang Fang's story "unacceptable" and I don't think any of them had to do with the "factual mistakes" included in the diary or reference to the "scandalous" photo of "abandoned cellphones." Those, I would argue, were the McGuffins introduced to distract readers from the real issues, which included a general tone that did not correspond to the political call for "positive energy" stories. Instead of cheerleading and singing the praises of the rapid construction of the Huoshenshan and Leishenshan Hospitals and other achievements lauded by state media, Fang Fang focused on how early announcements by heath officials that the virus was "Not Contagious Between People; It's Controllable and Preventable" (人不傳人、可防可控) had led to catastrophic consequences. In other words, instead of echoing the party-line line for "positive energy" narratives about the outbreak, Fang Fang openly criticized this form of didactic and propagandistic storytelling. This can be

---

[9] Hongwei Bao. "Three Woman and Their Wuhan Diaries: Women's Writing in a Quarantined Chinese City" October 17, 2020. Cha Journal. https://chajournal. blog/2020/10/17/wuhan-diaries/?fbclid=IwAR0Nj1WeJMcfA1ewUI729bIO9PQy74vO 7pX1W_dcAM_BooJ0gTcpk91GoBI

seen in Fang Fang's direct discussions of "positive energy," and open criticisms of internet censorship, and her forceful attack of the government's call for the citizens of Wuhan to express their "gratitude" towards the government. Guobin Yang has astutely observed that this "was surely the first time the ideology of positive energy was so directly and publicly challenged since its popularization in 2012. Fang Fang's challenge has a significance that goes beyond the immediate context."[10] But perhaps most damaging were Fang Fang's repeated calls for accountability. Throughout the diary, especially during the second half of her narrative, after the virus has been brought under control, Fang Fang emphasizes the need for accountability from local health officials and political leaders whose missteps, lack of action, and attempts to gag whistleblowers like Li Wenliang resulted in compounding the tragedy. Most of Fang Fang's calls for accountability were limited in scale and quite reasonable; but again, I would argue that the real perceived threat was with her readership. At the height of popularity, Fang Fang had tens of millions of loyal readers—even the thought of those readers being galvanized to demand accountability on other political issues would prove to be a threat with potentially destabilizing consequences. In other words, Fang Fang harnessed a "potential" that could not be tolerated. But it was not just the potential for amplification through readers that made Fang Fang's calls, as Guobin Yang described, it was "precisely because she is from within the establishment, her criticisms could be viewed as particularly hurtful and her calls for accountability especially threatening."[11]

Then there were other matters at stake that did not even exist when Fang Fang began writing her diary, but gradually came into play as the blog evolved. These issues included calls for international reparations from China for economic and other damages caused by COVID-19. These calls began quite early in the outbreak, with the International Council of Jurists, headquartered in London, who moved the UN Human Rights Council (UNHRC) to seek "unspecified reparations from China for having caused 'serious physical, psychological, economic and social harm' to

---

[10] Guobin Yang. *The Wuhan Lockdown*. New York: Columbia University Press: 2021. Pg. 151.
[11] Guobin Yang. *The Wuhan Lockdown*. New York: Columbia University Press: 2021. Pg. 151.

member-nations by unleashing Covid-19 on the world"[12] to claims made by US President Donald Trump that China will pay "big price" for the coronavirus on October 8, 2020.[13] The earliest of these calls for reparations began to gain headlines just days before news of the German and English translations of *Wuhan Diary* appeared on Chinese social media. A key part of the case for reparations lay rooted in providing evidence of "the origin of the virus." *Wuhan Diary* makes no mention of the reparations issue, nor does Fang Fang ever address the issue of COVID-19's origins; however, against the backdrop of these shifting political debates, Fang Fang's book was artificially pulled into these debates. Suddenly, in the eyes of Chinese ultra-nationalists, *Wuhan Diary* was going to provide "evidence" for the West on issues like reparations and the origins of the virus to use against China.

Playing into these fears, and certainly exacerbating them, were increasing political tensions between the United States and China. Naturally, the way in which *Wuhan Diary* became swept up in anti-American political rhetoric should not be looked at as an isolated case but as part of a pattern of anti-American political activism in China, which has intermittently swelled during times of crisis. With deep historical roots dating back to the "century of national humiliation" at the hands of Western powers, contemporary anti-American sentiment in the PRC came to a height during the Korean War with the "Resist America, Aid North Korea" movement. Of course, the Korean War was seven decades ago, but many of those same anti-American sentiments have been periodically tapped into since the launching of the Reform Era, from the anti-Spiritual Pollution campaign of 1983 and the 1989 Tiananmen crackdown, which can also be read as a rejection of Euro-American democratic ideals, to the 1999 US bombing of the Chinese embassy in Belgrade, which became a huge flashpoint in Sino-US relations and triggered massive waves of anti-American sentiment in China. Over the past 25 years, there have also been a series of bestselling Chinese books which have fanned the flames of anti-American sentiment, from *China Can Say No* to *Unhappy China* (*Zhongguo bu gaoxing* 中國不高興) and even to the numerous books praising Xi Jinping's

---

[12] A Subramani. "ICJ moves UNHRC against China for COVID-19 reparations" April 2, 2020 Times of India. https://timesofindia.indiatimes.com/india/icj-moves-unhcr-against-china-for-covid-19-reparations/articleshow/74965784.cms

[13] Joe Walsh. "Trump if Demanding China Pay 'Big Price' for Covid-19" October 8, 2020. Forbes. https://www.forbes.com/sites/joewalsh/2020/10/08/trump-is-demanding-china-pay-big-price-for-covid-19/#1faf5c5841c8

"Chinese Dream" (Zhongguo meng 中國夢), which can also be seen as a further rejection of American-style neoliberal ideals. The explosive anger articulated online over the American and German publication of *Wuhan Diary* must be contextualized within this complex history.

As Liao Guangsheng 廖光生 has observed, the foundation of Mao's anti-American theory was rooted in the "belief that imperialist power was shrinking while the power of the Chinese people was rising."[14] If we are to believe in this dialectical power relationship, it also says something about the current rise in anti-American sentiment surrounding *Wuhan Diary*. That is because as the attacks against the book were taking place, netizens were actively seeing the signs of China's "victory" over COVID-19, infection rates dripping, cities opening back up, life returning to normal, while, simultaneously, their screens were filled with signs of America's failure—social unrest tied to the killing of George Floyd, political chaos unleashed by the White House, widespread resistance to masks and lockdown policies, and rampant COVID-19 deaths. The long-slumbering anti-American discourse was not only resurrected, but it now finally appeared to be true. America seemed to be tearing itself apart from the inside just as Trump had decided on singling out China as his most consistent object of blame and ridicule. It was this dynamic which further reinforced the anti-American sentiment playing out throughout much of 2020.

As Donald Trump and members of his administration began labeling COVID-19 "the China virus" and "Kung Flu," news of the international publication of *Wuhan Diary* was repositioned as part of an "anti-China narrative" and Fang Fang's decision to proceed with publication was nothing less than an act of national betrayal. Within days, Fang Fang was one of the most popular searched terms on the Chinese internet, her name tied to a seemingly endless string of stories and posts about international reparations, the origin of the virus, and the US-China trade war, all topics she had never commented on and had had absolutely nothing to do with her diary. Like the Steven Spielberg film *Minority Report* where criminals are arrested and charged for "future crimes" that they are predicted to commit, in some sense, Fang Fang was the victim of a literary inquisition based on future crimes—that is, she "might" incite her broad readership to demand "accountability" from their government; *Wuhan Diary* "might" be used as a weapon by the West to hurt China. But none of these

---

[14] Liao Guangsheng 廖光生. *Exclusionism and Chinese Politics* (*Paiwai yu Zhongguo zhengzhi* 排外與中國政治). Taipei: Sanmin shuju, 1986. Pg. 136.

"crimes" ever came to pass. Donald Trump never held up *Wuhan Diary* during a White House press briefing and announced, "Here is the evidence!" In fact, the only place where these "crimes" occurred was in the posts of the Chinese trolls. However, after months of consistent messaging emanating from a network of disparate platforms—state media, social media posts, pop music, and cartoons—those "future crimes" became true for millions of Chinese internet users.

I would argue, however, that beyond debates about who gets to tell the story of the Wuhan outbreak and the myriad ways in which her book was artificially framed within the context of US-Chinese tensions, perhaps the single most explosive dimension of *Wuhan Diary* was its impact on larger debates concerning civil society in China. As attacks mounted and what had begun as a "controversy" evolved into a full-fledged "political incident" or what some critics characterized as an "online war,"[15] people began to position themselves along different political lines—those who felt Fang Fang had a right to publish her diary and express her opinions and those who felt she had crossed a line. Online and in living rooms all across China, intense debates broke out. Headlines with titles like "Has Fang Fang's Diary Ripped China Apart?!" (方方日記撕裂中國?!) and "Fang Fang's Diary and a Society Torn Apart" (方方日記與被撕裂的社會) began to appear. Many of Fang Fang's fans who supported her writings early on now felt that, by publishing *Wuhan Diary* abroad, an invisible line had been crossed; they felt that even if what she wrote was true, if the content of her book had a chance of harming the political or financial interests of the nation, it should be suppressed. Others stood by her, fervently fighting for Fang Fang's right to freely express her views and publish her diary. Others tried to take the middle ground; conservative editor of the party tabloid the *Global Times,* Hu Xijin harshly criticized the book, but at one point he did state that he "stands by the belief that Chinese society must tolerate the existence of Fang Fang's diary, which is a symbol

---

[15] Yang, Guobin. *The Wuhan Lockdown*. New York: Columbia University Press: 2021. Pg. 161. See also Lai Fu 來福. "The Battle Over Fang Fang: Old Answers and New Questions to the 'Theory of Passing the Knife'" (Fang Fang Zhanzheng: Tidaolun dejiuda'an he xin wenti 方方戰爭: 「剃刀論」的舊答案和新問題) Initium Media, May 20, 2020. https://theinitium.com/article/20200515-opinion-fangfang-people-war-national-socialism/ which refers to the "Battle Over Fang Fang" or "Fang Fang War."

of the most basic foundation of a pluralistic society,"[16] The rift around Fang Fang and her diary became so great that there were even mainstream news stories published that summarized which side of the political fence various writers and public intellectuals stood on the issue, with figures like Yi Zhongtian 易中天, Yan Lianke, Zhang Kangkang 張抗抗, and Zhu Dake on the pro-Fang Fang side and Hu Xijin, Zhang Yiwu, Zhang Hongliang, Wang Cheng, and Chen Xianyi 陳先義 on the detractors' team.[17] The debates of course, while superficially centered around *Wuhan Diary*, can be read more generally as a referendum on the state of civil society under Xi Jinping. Since roughly 2014, the space for free and open civil debate and artistic expression has been gradually shrinking. In fact, the deterioration of online discourse has been so severe that scholars Min Jiang and Ashley Esarey have characterized the rise of polarizing and hateful speech in China as "uncivil society."[18] The Fang Fang Incident harnessed several years of tensions about the future direction of civil society and online discourse in China, with one camp firmly supporting the CCP's hardline policies, which were viewed as an essential prerequisite for a prosperous society, and the other camp longing for a more open and transparent society where civil discourse, uncensored speech, and healthy debate can flourish. These tensions were, of course, further complicated and exacerbated by the spike in anti-Chinese political rhetoric originating from US politicians like Senator Marco Rubio and President Donald Trump during the early phase of the COVID-19 pandemic. The United States officially pivoting towards a harsher stance on China certainly played a crucial role in further polarizing Chinese netizens and turning even more people against *Wuhan Diary*, which trolls were actively aligning with the wave of anti-Chinese political discourse in the United States. *Wuhan Diary* became

---

[16] This is part of a statement Hu Xijin published on his Weibo account on April 9, 2020, at the height of the attacks on Fang Fang. The post was later reprinted online on numerous websites, including https://user.guancha.cn/main/content?id=283928.

[17] See for instance the article "Which celebrities publicly support Fang Fang" ("Na xie mingren gongkai zhichi Fang Fang?" 那些名人公開支持方方?) published on April 25, 2020, in China Business Focus (CBF): https://www.163.com/dy/article/FB28CPO4053770WR. html or the essay "Check Out Which Specialists Support Fang Fang and Who is Against Her" ("Kankan zhichi he fandui Fang Fang de zhuanjia dou you shei? 看看支持和反對方方的專家都有誰?) by Feng Yunkan https://zhuanlan.zhihu.com/p/133760882.

[18] For more on the concept of "uncivil society," see Min Jiang and Ashley Esarey, "Uncivil Society in Digital Society: Incivility, Fragmentation, and Political Stability" in *International Journal of Communication*. Vol 12 (2018). https://ijoc.org/index.php/ijoc/article/view/9478/2340.

a lightning rod for many issues, but its role in inspiring a new debate about civil society in China may be one of its most important lasting legacies.

The heated discussions about *Wuhan Diary* also spun off into the field of law as a deluge of legal debates began to appear online. One by one, armchair lawyers and bona fide legal specialists began to weigh in on everything from the chances of Fang Fang winning a libel case against her detractors to why the state had still not arrested her on charges of subversion or treason. The legal debates began on April 9, 2020, exactly when the deluge of troll attacks started online, and it is difficult not to read them side by side. One headline from that date read "Is Everything in Fang Fang's Diary True? If Not, What Legal and Moral Responsibility Should She Carry?". In that article the author concluded that although "it would be extremely difficult to hold her accountable legally…from the perspective of moral responsibility, Fang Fang had already committed an act of betrayal. She now has a cangue around her neck and there was no way for her to escape."[19] But that was just the beginning; over the ensuing months questions surrounding Fang Fang's crime and punishment would inundate the Chinese internet and grow more heated and accusatory over time. Articles like "Do you feel like Fang Fang already broke the law? Do you support her being prosecuted to the fullest extent of the law?" (你認為方方已經觸犯法律嗎?你支持起訴方方將其繩之以法嗎?) and "Ten Basic Legal Questions Raised by the Fang Fang Diary Phenomena" (方方日記現象涉及的十個基本法律問題)[20] went viral and further fueled the more general debates raging about the diary. It is interesting that the majority of the articles were published under pseudonyms (or simply without a byline) and were framed as questions, as if the authors themselves were afraid of being tried for libel. One essay published on July 8, 2020, entitled "Why is Fang Fang So Blind? Will She Face Legal Censure?" stated:

> Fang Fang's writing is something that is not even worth mentioning, but by taking a personal record and calling it "Wuhan Diary" and even selling it in

[19] Eagle in the Sky天空中的鷹, "Is Everything in Fang Fang's Diary True? If Not, What Legal and Moral Responsibility Should She Carry?" (方方日記寫的都是事實嗎?如果不是她應負什麼法律和道義責任?) http://qdcypf.com/q-201810.html

[20] The ten basic legal questions cited in Yidizaiyaogong's latter article include questions concerning (1) constitutional rights, (2) the responsibility of international law, (3) criminal law (including corruption, slander, and death threats), (4) administrative illegalities, (5) private business law, and (6) how to settle online disputes. For more see https://zhuanlan.zhihu.com/p/129808349.

the name of a series of "dispatches" is completely wrong. This falls under the umbrella of intentionally deceiving readers in order to attain personal profit and fame; it is clearly illegal. But as for whether or not legal codes will be enforced to carry out serious punishment against her, we will have to wait and see how the nation responds![21]

It was as if alongside the academic and pop culture attacks, a series of legal arguments were being methodically built up and projected into the public sphere in order to justify and rationalize the ongoing attacks.

Unfortunately, in the short term at least, the way in which COVID-19 has played out seems to have worked in favor of the trolls. As COVID-19 cases continued to escalate throughout North America and Europe, China began to reopen and get its society and economy back on track. As, one after another, Western nations faltered in their handling of the novel coronavirus outbreak, the Chinese model gained newfound support among its citizens. In the wake of the Chinese "victory" over the virus, not only have Fang Fang's early calls for "accountability" been forgotten, but, in the eyes of her detractors, the campaign against her has been justified. In the eyes of her detractors, with the West's failure to control COVID-19 throughout 2020, the more liberal, Western, and democratic-leaning ideas that Fang Fang's diary seems to represent have been "proven" inferior to Xi Jinping's hardline authoritarian principles.

Given the tenacity and protracted nature of the attacks, I have been repeatedly asked why Fang Fang was never arrested. After all, there were a group of independent journalists and bloggers like Chen Qiushi 陳秋實, Fang Bin方斌, Li Zehua 李澤華, and Zhang Zhan 張展 who "disappeared" while reporting on the Wuhan outbreak.[22] And according to journalist Jasper Becker:

> More than 5,100 people in China were arrested for sharing information in the first weeks of the outbreak. Dissidents were labelled as sick, so the government could place them in medical quarantine. Hundreds of ordinary

---

[21] Little Tiger Has Something to Say 小虎有話說 "Why is Fang Fang So Blind? Will She Face Legal Censure?" (方方為什至今執迷不悔，她會不會受到法律的制裁?) http://www.yidianzixun.com/article/0PoUkkRM

[22] Rosie Perper "A 4th Chinese citizen journalist was reportedly detained while livestreaming what life was like in Wuhan at the height of the coronavirus outbreak." May 18, 2020 Business Insider. https://www.businessinsider.com/zhang-zhan-fourth-chinese-journalist-arrested-for-livestreaming-in-wuhan-2020-5

citizens were detained and fined over innocuous online messages over hospital queues, mask shortages, and the death of relatives.[23]

I should confess that, throughout the period I was translating *Wuhan Diary* and as the attacks were raging online, my single greatest fear was that something might happen to Fang Fang. Given the unprecedented nature of the attacks, the death threats, bricks thrown over the wall of her residence, denunciation posters appearing around her house, public calls for her to be tried for treason, and widespread censure she was facing, I don't think my fears were unfounded. Those fears kept me up at night. My agent and I had numerous conversations about what we could do to help ensure her safety; but we were also struck by a sense of helplessness. Meanwhile, whenever Fang Fang spoke publicly of the threats, her detractors just claimed she was just trying to exploit her misery to gain sympathy from the public.[24] But there were a few factors that provided some level of protection for Fang Fang. Firstly, unlike the independent journalists who were detained in Wuhan, Fang Fang was not a dissident or an activist. She is a heavily decorated veteran writer who served as head of the Hubei Writers Association, a title which certainly provided some level of protection. But more than that was the wellspring of public support she had nurtured over the **60** days during which she wrote her diary. The diary had arguably given Fang Fang the broadest readership she had ever enjoyed over the course of her career; that readership, who waited up every night for her next diary installment, also provided a layer of protection. Persecuting a writer who had been regarded as "the voice of Wuhan" could easily backfire. This lesson became particularly apparent in the wake of Li Wenliang's death. After Li's death there was a palatable mood of anger and resentment in the air; the outpouring of public support for Li was so great that the government was forced to suddenly offer a political reappraisal of his actions and posthumously declare him a martyr in the fight against COVID-19. But I suspect his death also provided an added layer of defense for Fang Fang. Having just felt the sting of the public's collective wrath over how Li was treated, the last thing the government

---

[23] Becker, Jasper. *Made in China: Wuhan, COVID and the Quest for Biotech Supremacy.* London: C. Hurst & Co. 2021. Pg. 267.

[24] In Fang Fang's "About" series she would later devote an entire installment to these claims she was "exploiting her misery." See "About: Exploiting Misery" ("Guanyu: Maican" 關於：賣慘) originally published on WeChat and reposted on Radio France International: https://www.rfi.fr/cn/中国/20200505-方方-关于-5-关于卖惨.

would want to do would be to incite the public's ire over Fang Fang. At the same time, Fang Fang was a problem. The previously outlined concerns about her book were real; yet she hadn't really "done anything wrong." In this sense, the question of how to deal with Fang Fang became a difficult quandary for the powers that be. She would not relent or give in to political pressure and refused to cancel international publication plans for her book. And so, other methods were employed; trolls were released and allowed to roam free throughout their virtual online kingdom, spreading lies, making threats, discrediting the author, wreaking havoc, and, gradually, changing the public's perception of *Wuhan Diary*.

Delving deep into this anatomy of a Chinese cyber disinformation campaign, one can see patterns of mutual reinforcement. Both official media articles and posts from influential "VIP" users on Weibo with millions of followers inspire large numbers of individual trolls (which include both paid members of the so-called 50 Cent Army and netizens motivated by anger and genuine feelings of nationalism); meanwhile academic scholar-trolls like Zhang Yiwu endorsed pop culture commentaries like Wuheqilin (the artist behind "Crown a Jester"), who is further legitimized through official state media portals like the *Global Times*. While, on the surface, these different levels of attacks—nationalistic individuals, paid trolls, academic detractors, official media reports, armchair lawyers citing legal code violations, and pop culture interventions—seem completely separate, giving the illusion of an organic, grassroots movement, they are in fact connected through a deep network of mutual reinforcement and legitimization. Moreover, they collectively converge to form what I would argue is the illusion of a mass culture consensus. This mass culture consensus refers to a concerted effort aimed at presenting a unified system of messaging across different platforms that seems to simultaneously represent high culture and low culture as well as both official and non-official discourse, whereas, in reality, they are all working in coordination to present a unified ideological vision. In the case of *Wuhan Diary*, rap songs ("Literary Scum") and political cartoons ("Crown a Jester") seem to represent low culture, pseudo-academic books (*Great Wuhan But Bad Diary*) represent high culture, official media outlets (the *Global Times*, China Military) voice the opinion of the state, and online trolls seem to present an edgier non-official discourse; in reality, they are all part of a hegemonic process of mutual reinforcement that forces a single perspective down multiple channels of expression. Netizens trying to navigate this illusion of mass culture consensus are in a particularly precarious position; they are flooded with a single ideological message dressed up in a multitude of guises; meanwhile, alternative perspectives and voices are systematically silenced. It is this convergence that poses the greatest threat to the democratization of ideas, an open public sphere, and the very existence of a civil society

Although this is a case study of a single Chinese disinformation campaign, it is very much a harbinger of a much broader global threat. The global dimension of the threat is not just the implication of Chinese trolls "spilling over" from behind the Great Firewall and attempting to influence discourse on Facebook, Twitter, Amazon, and other foreign websites, but even more terrifying is the ubiquitous nature of the threat. The campaign against *Wuhan Diary* is quite similar to disinformation campaigns being launched right here in the United States and in countries all over the world. While both the Democratic and Republican parties seem superficially united in their criticism of many of Xi Jinping's policies, in reality, their own policies in the United States have created a cyber environment wherein identical policies of fake news, disinformation, online political manipulation, and "manufactured consensus" are being actively practiced right here at home.

CHAPTER 11

Lessons

Over the course of translating *Wuhan Diary* and, later, writing this book, there were several times that I was struck by an unsettling feeling that something was lost. Fang Fang's diary is, in many ways, a book about the most fundamental questions of life and death, and yet the internet was alit with thousands of petty attacks strangely fixated upon the most trivial and mundane of details—did Fang Fang fabricate a photograph of orphaned cellphones? Did she misreport details concerning a nurse's death? *Wuhan Diary* is a book depicting an existential struggle, a portrait of a city and her people during their darkest hour as they faced an invisible threat that everyone was still grappling to understand; yet a strategy of distraction seemed to dictate so much of the public discourse surrounding the book. The odd thing was that, somehow, as the petty microscope of the internet trolls tried to repeatedly bring the public's attention to the most insignificant of details, the book and the attacks themselves were simultaneously tapping into one of the biggest issues of our current historical era—the COVID-19 pandemic, diplomatic tensions between China and the West, fake news, cyber-attack campaigns, the manipulation of social media, and the global rise of authoritarianism. It is a strange confluence, a mismatched overlap that feels surreal, almost blasphemous, and yet it also, in some sense, captures the unusual tone of the diary itself, which vacillates between chronicles of the quotidian and encounters with the epic.

M. Berry, *Translation, Disinformation, and Wuhan Diary*,
https://doi.org/10.1007/978-3-031-16859-8_11

Even over the very short period of time since its initial posting and publication in book form, *Wuhan Diary* is a text whose meaning has continued to transform over time. Initially I thought I was translating a book about a virus; it turned out to be much more than that. In my 2008 book *A History of Pain: Trauma in Chinese Literature and Film* I pinpointed two different modes through which trauma has been processed through the dual lenses of culture and politics: centripetal trauma and centrifugal trauma. Centripetal trauma refers to traumatic events whose "origins lie on the outside" yet "they often inspire a renewed examination or articulation of the Chinese nation"[1]—the rise of nationalist sentiment in China during the wake of events ranging from the Second Sino-Japanese War (1937–1945) to the 1999 US bombing of the Chinese embassy in Belgrade which are both good examples of centripetal trauma—whereas centrifugal trauma "is used to describe a radical shift in the creation of traumatic narratives, which are introduced from within, generated in the center, and projected outward…."[2] This outward projection alternately triggers cycles of destabilization, disillusionment, and diasporic impulses; think of the wave of Chinese students and intellectuals who fled abroad in the wake of the 1989 Tiananmen massacre as a representative case. These are not always "clean-cut" processes; there often exist tensions and inter-bleeding between these two modes. But I know of almost no other examples where a single text went from being clearly defined and framed in one category before morphing into the other in just a matter of days. In the case of *Wuhan Diary*, the blog in its initial form and reception can be read as an example of centrifugal trauma: it was a portrait of an internal crisis, and the many accounts of prejudice against Hubei residents, lack of access to medical care and hospital beds, and failure on the part of local leaders all pointed to a process of destabilization, and a thrust beginning at a single epicenter—Wuhan—and reverberating outward. That outward thrust can be seen in the cries of the sick begging for medical care and Fang Fang's calls for accountability and perhaps most palpably felt in the broad outrage after the death of Li Wenliang. In fact, I would argue that this centrifugal movement can be seen not only in *Wuhan Diary*, but also in society as a whole, at least during the early phase of the outbreak in Wuhan. However, sensing the

---

[1] Berry, Michael. *A History of Pain: Trauma in Modern Chinese Literature and Film.* New York: Columbia University Press, 2008. Pg. 5.
[2] Ibid. Pg. 6.

danger of these destabilizing effects, a campaign was swiftly implemented to change the course of how the outbreak was imagined and perceived and, in the process, also transform public discourse around both *Wuhan Diary* and the coronavirus outbreak itself. From January to April of 2020 conspiracy theories that attributed "more responsibility to the United States than to China" began to inundate Weibo.[3] Fang Fang came under attack, her supporters were silenced, national narratives of "victory" drowned out earlier calls for accountability, and the United States entered the conversation as an aggressor: Chinese Foreign Ministry spokesman Zhao Lijian, adopting a new Wolf Warrior tone, suggested that the US Army had smuggled the virus into Wuhan[4] and later various media outlets in China suggested that the foreign publication of *Wuhan Diary* was interpreted as an act of aggression against China—these moves, and others like them, introduced an external aggressor into the coronavirus story. Suddenly, what had been an internal trauma was now repackaged and redefined as an example of centripetal trauma, an attack from the outside that would trigger an unprecedented nationalistic response, a new tide of anti-American activism, and transform the COVID-19 outbreak into a patriotic call to arms. As Zheng Wang has observed, "Chinese nationalism has long proved to be an extremely effective device for providing a sense of solidarity in times of social unrest and political uncertainty."[5] As US-China diplomatic relations became more strained, Chinese nationalism surged and a hate campaign was harnessed against the diary that had dared to ask questions and call for accountability. Along the way, Fang Fang's poetry, *When an era sheds a speck of dust it might not seem like much, but when it falls upon the shoulders of an individual it feels like a mountain*—words that had once captured the hearts of millions of Chinese readers at the start of the pandemic—had been erased.

Part of the changing meaning of *Wuhan Diary* over time lies in the new lessons that I have continued to take away from Fang Fang. Over the course

---

[3] Kaiping Chen, Anfan Chen, Jingwen Zhang, Jingbo Meng, and Cuihua Shen. "Conspiracy and debunking narratives about COVID-19 origins on Chinese social media: How it started and who is to blame" *Misinformation Review*. December 10, 2020. https://misinforeview.hks.harvard.edu/article/conspiracy-and-debunking-narratives-about-covid-19-origins-on-chinese-social-media-how-it-started-and-who-is-to-blame/

[4] https://www.latimes.com/world-nation/story/2020-05-04/wolf-warrior-diplomats-defend-china-handling-coronavirus

[5] Wang, Zheng. *Never Forget National Humiliation: Historical Memory in Chinese Politics and Foreign Relations*. New York: Columbia University Press, 2012. Pg. 228.

of its 60 entries, *Wuhan Diary* contained only a handful of minor references to the United States—news of a Chinese-American artist who donated to Wuhan, mention of PPE and other medical supplies donated by the city of Pittsburgh, or mention of Fang Fang's old classmate, Old Fox, who once walked the Appalachian Trail—yet somehow the book played directly into the hands of the trade war and the unfolding tensions in US-China diplomatic relations. The book was positioned within Chinese online discourse as part of a scheme to harm the Chinese nation; Fang Fang and even I as the translator were both characterized as agents for the CIA, and the book was leveraged as a political instrument during a time of unprecedented tension between the US and China. This meant that the cyber campaign against the book took on a distinctly transpacific context, which was fueled by COVID-19's early potentially destabilizing impact upon domestic politics and a global rise in anti-Chinese sentiment. This meant that the cyber response would not only prominently address the global dimension through rhetoric aimed at Chinese netizens, but also attempt to directly target overseas internet users (through platforms like Twitter and Amazon) in shaping how discourse around the book was shaped globally. Yet if we strip away all the controversy, attacks, and cyber noise circulating around the book, there are key lessons to be learned from *Wuhan Diary*. Many of these are highly personal lessons, and since this began as a personal story perhaps it is appropriate that this is how the story ends. Several of these lessons also address the United States, as the campaign against *Wuhan Diary* was always deeply rooted in the vicious cycle of political antagonism playing out between China and the US during 2020.

Earlier I discussed *Wuhan Diary* in relation to Lu Xun's iconic short story "A Madman's Diary." In some sense, *Wuhan Diary* is a real-life cry from an "iron house." A desperate attempt to shake the bars and scream aloud, hoping to wake up a long-slumbering nation. In that sense, Fang Fang is firmly positioned in a literary tradition that goes from Lu Xun's *Call to Arms* (*Nahan* 吶喊) to Bo Yang's 柏楊 *The Ugly Chinaman* (*Chouluo de Zhongguo ren* 醜陋的中國人) to Lung Yingtai's 龍應台 *Wildfire* (*Yehuo ji* 野火集). While those earlier examples all took aim at the Chinese cultural and historical tradition, in 2020, as COVID-19 transformed into a global pandemic, Fang Fang's *Wuhan Diary* would prove to be prescient for people around the world as the virus spread. Some of Fang Fang's lessons had to do with simple and practical public health measures, others had to do with the virus of disinformation and fake news, while further lessons touched on deeper issues regarding the nature of civil society.

Lesson #1, Public Health Protocols. One of the most divisive aspects of the COVID-19 health crisis has been the different public health policies that various regions have adopted in terms of how to manage the pandemic. Local policies have elicited radically different responses both among the constituents whom those policies directly effect and internationally, in terms of how those polices are endorsed or criticized. As the first city-wide lockdown of the COVID-19 era, the Wuhan lockdown also took on a highly politicized tone. *Time* magazine called the lockdown "draconian";[6] Yanzhong Huang from Council on Foreign Relations was quoted in *The Washington Post* as saying, "only the Chinese government could implement draconian measures to such a large scale."[7] Human Rights Watch claimed "authorities failed to ensure appropriate access to medical, food, and other necessities."[8] Meanwhile, in China the lockdown was largely praised by official state media for its "effectiveness." At the same time, private responses varied widely: the majority of citizens steadfastly supported government policies, while there also existed widespread sentiments of anger and frustration, especially as the Wuhan lockdown extended to a full 76 days. Two years later, when Xi'an, Shanghai, and other cities in China also experienced strict extended lockdowns, the public response began to transform: while most begrudgingly cooperated an undercurrent of frustration and unrest was also captured in remarkable moments, such as the short six-minute video Voice of April (Siyue zhi sheng 四月之聲), which went viral on Chinese social on April 22, 2022. Later as many other nations around the world instituted their own versions of lockdowns, or stay-at-home orders, they also faced varying degrees of cooperation and blowback. This mixed response extended not only to lockdowns, but other COVID-19-related policies relating to face masks social distancing, and vaccines.

Three years into the pandemic, it is instructive to look back to see what we can learn from Fang Fang in terms of public health policies. According to Fang Fang's account, she first wore a face mask on January 18, 2020, when she visited a friend in the hospital. At the time, there were still no official announcements about an outbreak, yet in response to rumors of a

[6] Amy Gunia. "China's Draconian Lockdown Is Getting Credit for Slowing Coronavirus. Would It Work Anywhere Else?" *Time* March 13, 2020. https://time.com/5796425/china-coronavirus-lockdown/

[7] Siobhan O'Grady. "China's coronavirus lockdown—brought to you by authoritarianism" The Washington Post. January 27, 2020. https://www.washingtonpost.com/world/2020/01/27/chinas-coronavirus-lockdown-brought-you-by-authoritarianism/

[8] "China: Events of 2020" https://www.hrw.org/world-report/2021/country-chapters/china-and-tibet#

new SARS-like illness spreading in Wuhan, Fang Fang began to don a mask. At the time, there was very little information about what this virus was, how it spread, and who was at risk, yet, out of an overabundance of caution, Fang Fang begins wearing a mask. Compare that to so many Western nations that failed to initially adopt mask mandates (in the United States, the government did not issue a nationwide mask mandate until President Joe Biden took office a full year after the start of the pandemic), and even after mandates were imposed we even witnessed the absurd rise of the "anti-masker movements" in countries around the world.

Fang Fang also took a similar stance on the quarantine measures. Wuhan's lockdown began on January 23 and lasted until April 8, lasting a total of 76 days. At the time, the length and severity of the lockdown was unprecedented. Residents were quarantined inside their homes and required to have regular temperature checks, and food shopping was strictly regulated, yet, as Fang Fang observed, "Wuhan's nine million residents worked together to cooperate with all the government's requests; their restraint and patience helped to ensure that Wuhan would be able to contain this virus...."[9] Wuhan was able to effectively control the outbreak and the city was able to open back up in April of 2020. Compare that to countries like the United States, the United Kingdom, and Brazil where government officials initially downplayed the virus. Even though countries like China and Italy took the brunt of the initial outbreak, buying time for other nations to prepare, crucial time was squandered and no national policies were implemented. In the United States individual states were left on their own to devise stay-at-home orders, and, even when such policies were adopted, large segments of the population chose not to cooperate with basic guidelines put forth by public health specialists.

The deep disparity on this issue is laid naked by juxtaposing Fang Fang's comments on mass gatherings with the US administration's actions. On January 20, even before the city of Wuhan enacted its lockdown, Fang Fang wrote:

> I think that the community deciding to move forward with this large-scale gathering while this "new virus" is still spreading is basically a form of criminal action. No matter how much you love showing off for the leaders or how much you love displaying the power of this great era of peace and

---

[9] Fang Fang. *Wuhan Diary: Dispatches from a Quarantined City*. New York: HarperVia, 2020. Pg. xiv.

prosperity, for the time being the municipal government should ban all large-scale public gatherings like this; even if the participants are willing to take the risk, the government should still step in and prevent them from doing so.[10]

As I translated this and other passages from Fang Fang's diary in March, Donald Trump was still insisting on holding mass political rallies throughout the country: the White House hosted a super spreader event at the Rose Garden on September 26, 2020, and even as late as October 2020, Donald Trump was still hosting large unmasked rallies. Time and time again, the United States put "displays of power" and its love of "showing off its leaders" above the health and safety of its citizens. When Fang Fang was offering her scathing criticism back in January 2020, few people understood how COVID-19 was transmitted or how truly serious it could be. This is not to defend those early public gatherings that took place in Wuhan, but, at the very least, that was during the early phase of this pandemic where there was so little understanding and good science to base assessments on. What was the United States' excuse?

While Fang Fang repeatedly encouraged her readers to comply with the government's lockdown policies and emphasized her support, there were limits to said support. As the lockdown dragged on and positive case numbers in Wuhan began to radically decline, Fang Fang began openly calling for the city to open up again. She also repeatedly offered suggestions through her blog to help solve some of the medical problems the city was facing during the height of the COVID-19 crisis, such as her February 2 and 14 discussions of busing patients in dire need of non-COVID medical intervention out of the city to hospitals in neighboring provinces. Thus while Fang Fang overall offered strong and consistent support of her government's major policies, she also offered constructive suggestions, pragmatic calls to loosen internet censorship restrictions, and openly expressed her frustration as the lockdown extended past the two-month mark. This points to an approach rooted in flexible compliance with government policies but also deeply informed by her own self-education in the latest medical knowledge and on-the-ground situation in hospitals regarding infection numbers and availability of hospital beds. Given the early crackdown on whistleblowers in Wuhan and lack of transparency concerning the

---

[10] Ibid. Pg. 224.

infectiousness of the novel coronavirus, Fang Fang seemed intent on personally arming herself with the latest information in order to make informed decisions.

Internationally, we saw different forms of policy failures, misguided medical advice, and the use of disinformation in how various governments approached local COVID-19 outbreaks. Take for instance early CDC guidelines in the United States that face masks were not needed. On February 29, 2020, US Surgeon General Dr. Jerome Adams sent out an official tweet that read: "Seriously people—STOP BUYING MASKS! They are NOT effective in preventing general public from catching #Coronavirus, but if healthcare providers can't get them to care for sick patients, it puts them and our communities at risk!"[11] Of course, we know in hindsight that this type of messaging was aimed at addressing a severe shortage of masks and other PPE during the early pandemic, but it also severely compromised citizens' trust in the government. This was not dissimilar to the impact Wuhan-based public health officials that claimed person-to-person transmission was not possible had on public trust in government. (In the United States, it could also be argued that early discouragement of face masks also helped set in motion the later anti-masker movement.) Returning to Fang Fang, who did not base her decision to wear a face mask on January 18 on government protocols (none were in place at that time), but on *common sense* safety protocols, what emerges as an important takeaway in terms of the need for citizens to self-educate and make personal healthcare decisions based on science-based data and resist blind endorsement of public health policies that are driven by politics instead of science? (Think of how Fang Fang largely supported the government's lockdown policies because they made sense from a public health perspective, but strongly resisted the government's call for Wuhan citizens to express the "gratitude" to the Chinese Communist Party, as it was purely politically motivated.) In retrospect, Fang Fang's urge to de-couple politics from public health is an important takeaway as countries around the world continue to grapple with the deeply entrenched politicization of COVID-19 messaging and related healthcare policies.

Lesson #2, Civil Society. Just as *Wuhan Diary* triggered a widespread debate in China about the core nature, functions, and responsibilities of

---

[11] Deborah Netburn. "A Timeline of the CDC's advice on facemasks" July 27, 2021. Los Angeles Times. https://www.latimes.com/science/story/2021-07-27/timeline-cdc-mask-guidance-during-covid-19-pandemic

civil society, so too those lessons resonate globally, especially in the United States. Just as the diary tapped into a deep political fissure running through Chinese society, so too 2020 has marked a year of unprecedented political divide and turmoil in the United States. The COVID-19 era may have marked the beginning of a new period of heightened diplomatic tension between the United States and China; however, after living in the shadow of *Wuhan Diary* and the fallout around the book, I became increasingly haunted by the uncanny similarities with the United States that continued to appear. As the COVID-19 outbreak spread unchecked and the death toll in the United States climbed, Yam Bear Six along with countless other trolls in China began to taunt me online: "Write your American Diary! You fascist extremist!"

In one of her most remarkable diary entries, on March 7, Fang Fang recorded her shock, anger, and appalment at the call for citizens to express their "gratitude" to the government for its handling of the coronavirus outbreak. An incensed Fang Fang instead called for the government to own up to its missteps.

> ...My dear government, please suck in your pride and humbly extend your gratitude to your masters—the millions of citizens of Wuhan.
>
> Next the government should make haste and beg for the people's forgiveness. This is the time for reflection and assuming responsibility. A rational government with a conscience that listens to the needs of its people and understands how to console them should, at this very moment, quickly establish an independent investigative team to piece together the full details surrounding the outbreak, who was responsible for delaying the response, who decided to withhold information about the outbreak from the public, who were the leaders that in order to save face decided to twist the truth when reporting to their superiors and hide the truth from the public, who was it who put political correctness above the lives of our people, how many people contributed to this disaster? Whoever had a hand in this should take responsibility; the people need someone to assume accountability. At the same time, the government should urge officials from various departments whose actions misguided the public, leading to massive numbers of deaths, to resign. Individuals to be investigated should include high-level government administrators, top officials from the Ministry of Propaganda, those in the media who helped cover things up, and top officials from the Department of Health. If any of them are criminally liable, let the courts decide their punishment. However, based on my observations, most Chinese government officials are lacking when it comes to self-reflection, not to mention

those willing to take the blame and resign. In a situation like this, citizens should, at the very least, draft a public call for all those officials who took politics as the center of their world while treating people like trash to resign. How can we let these people with blood on their hands continue strutting around in front of the people of Wuhan, gesticulating as if they are heroes? Supposing that 10 or 20 officials stand up and resign as a result of this, at least we will know that there are at least a few officials left who still have a conscience.[12]

While Fang Fang expressed her outrage at the Chinese government's self-congratulatory gestures and celebratory cries of "victory," at the very least, China seemed to have turned a corner in its efforts to contain COVID-19. Meanwhile in the United States, as the virus spread and deaths mounted, the US government had already begun its own (premature) victory march. An April 16, 2020, article in Vox quoted Donald Trump's comments that the United States has "more or less declared victory over the coronavirus during the daily White House briefing."[13] Then on May 8, 2020, *The Philadelphia Tribune* published an article entitled "Trump declares victory as virus death toll rises."[14] On May 12, 2020, *Australian Financial Review* published the article "Trump declares victory over the virus," which described how "President Trump declared America has 'met the moment and we have prevailed' by delivering a testing capacity that is 'unmatched and unrivalled anywhere in the world.'"[15] Fang Fang expressed disgust when the Chinese government declared "victory" against the virus when new infection rates dropped down to the single digits. The point being that there is no "winner," after suffering thousands of deaths, there is nothing to "celebrate"; it is instead a time for reflection, remembrance, and mourning. But how do we make sense of Donald Trump's declarations of "victory" even as the COVID-19 death

[12] Fang Fang. *Wuhan Diary: Dispatches from a Quarantined City*. New York: HarperVia, 2020. Pg. 235–236.

[13] "Trump just declared victory over the coronavirus. Here's why that's premature." In Vox, April 16, 2020. https://www.vox.com/2020/4/16/21224405/opening-up-america-again-trump-coronavirus-testing

[14] "Trump declares victory as virus death toll rises" in The Philadelphia Tribune, May 8, 2020. https://www.phillytrib.com/news/health/coronavirus/trump-declares-victory-as-virus-death-toll-rises/article_b72114f6-9245-5ab2-ab80-bd780384c2b7.html

[15] "Trump declares victory over the virus" in Australian Financial Review, May 12, 2020. https://www.afr.com/world/north-america/us-crawls-back-to-work-white-house-orders-staff-wear-masks-20200512-p54s0r

rates and infection numbers were continuing to soar? What does it say about the United States as a nation?

There has been widespread coverage about the worldwide spike of anti-Chinese and anti-Asian racism since the COVID-19 outbreak began. *Wuhan Diary*'s detractors even argued that the book would fuel discrimination and acts of racist violence. In reality, long before Trump started referring to COVID-19 as the "China Virus" or "Kung Flu," fueling anti-Chinese sentiment in the United States, there had actually been a similar dynamic playing out on a micro-level in China itself. Fang Fang had actually described how the virus had fueled discrimination against people from Wuhan in her very first diary entry: "What happened led Wuhan to become the focal point of the entire nation, it led to the city being locked down, the people of Wuhan being subjected to prejudice...."[16] Whereas Fang Fang identified how discrimination and racism have been tied to the virus from the very beginning, political leaders in the United States have continued to take actions and make statements that directly fuel and incite racism, reinforcing damaging rhetoric that conflates race with disease. As Trump and key members of his regime, including Mike Pompeo and Peter Navarro, continued to publicly denigrate China, they simultaneously fell into the same pitfalls that Fang Fang had warned us about in the Chinese government's handling of the outbreak, including the provincialization and politicization of the virus. As forces in China worked to actively suppress the publication of *Wuhan Diary* both in China and abroad, we saw the Trump regime, one after another, file multiple lawsuits in an attempt to suppress the publication of books by Mary Trump, Michael Cohen, and John Bolton. And as online trolls in China accused Fang Fang of being a "spy" or a "secret agent" and carried out a witch hunt against her supporters, similar forces were also taking shape in the United States. The US government formally accused US-based academics like Anming Hu (University of Tennessee) and Gang Chen (MIT) as "spies," charges which were eventually dismissed or proven to be erroneous.[17] After Donald

---

[16] Fang Fang. *Wuhan Diary: Dispatches from a Quarantined City*. New York: HarperVia, 2020. Pg. 3.

[17] See for instance: Joe Saballa. "UT Faculty Calls to Reinstate Prof Accused of Being a Spy" *The College Post*. October 4, 2021. https://thecollegepost.com/ut-faculty-calls-to-reinstate-prof-accused-of-being-chinese-spy/ And Ellen Nakashima. "Charges dismissed against MIT professor accused of hiding research ties to China." *The Washington Post*. January 20, 2022. https://www.washingtonpost.com/national-security/mit-gang-chen-dismiss/2022/01/20/912f68aa-786b-11ec-bf97-6eac6f77fba2_story.html.

Trump fired Secretary of Defense Mark Esper in November 2020, the White House "reportedly demanded a list of names of people who clapped as [Esper] left the building."[18] Just as Chinese netizens were having their own debate about the nature of civil society and whether they wanted an online environment that persecuted people for supporting a woman's right to publish a diary, so too the United States needs to reflect on whether we want a society that attempts to persecute individuals simply for clapping out an ousted colleague and attempts to suppress unflattering political biographies. The very Chinese authoritarian policies and practices that the Trump White House railed against in public statements (no doubt to distract American citizens from their own failures) were, in fact, becoming increasingly manifest in everyday US political policies.

Lesson # 3: Disinformation. The controversy surrounding *Wuhan Diary* provided a dark glimpse into the power that disinformation wields in undermining iconoclastic voices and reinforcing "the good story of China." Throughout *Wuhan Diary* and its account of the COVID-19 outbreak runs the parallel narrative of disinformation, fake news, and cyber-politics. Fang Fang first mentioned the troll attacks in her February 13 entry, about one quarter into the diary, but as the narrative continued, engagement with online politics became an increasingly prominent facet of the book. Ultimately, the attacks became so frequent that they almost seemed to eclipse the threat of COVID-19. Fang Fang even reserved the final entry of *Wuhan Diary* to launch a scathing statement of censure and warning against the damaging impact of the rising culture of disinformation, trolls, and online hate:

> The presence of these ultra-leftists represents an existential threat to China and her people! They are the greatest hindrance to the Reform Era! If we allow the ultra-leftists to throw their weight around as they wish and spread their disease throughout our society, the reforms will die, and China's future will be doomed.[19]

---

[18] Alexander, Harriet. "White House 'requesting names of those who clapped out departing Pentagon official'" November 12, 2020. The Independent: https://www.independent.co.uk/news/world/americas/us-election-2020/white-house-department-of-defense--pentagon-jim-anderson-b1721307.html

[19] Fang Fang. *Wuhan Diary: Dispatches from a Quarantined City.* New York: HarperVia, 2020. Pg. 354.

While some may write off online trolls as a fringe group with limited influence, these are powerful words that testify to the deeply destructive power these forces wield and the threat they pose to civil society. In some sense, Fang Fang bearing witness to these voices which rose up to infect Weibo, WeChat, and other social media platforms was just as important as her record of the coronavirus outbreak. However just as the coronavirus knows no boundaries, so too the viral online attacks and disinformation campaigns also are not limited to China. As the ultra-leftists attacked Fang Fang and countless other figures in China, here in the United States a parallel virus was taking root. Driven by radical nationalist ideology, conspiracy theories, seemingly ubiquitous political lies, a distrust of truth (which is labeled "fake news"), and a violent social media sphere spearheaded by the alt-right and related groups, America in 2020 also became a land of trolls.

Spending 2020 immersed in translating *Wuhan Diary* and the ensuing controversies surrounding the book on Chinese social media, the similarities between the Chinese ultra-leftists and the American alt-right were startling. Some of these parallels include (1) embracing an extremist nationalist and anti-foreign agenda; (2) looking to darker historical periods for inspiration and legitimation (the Jim Crow era of the American South or Nazi Germany for the US alt-right and the Cultural Revolution for the Chinese ultra-left); (3) tapping into a collective nostalgia for a time when now disenfranchised classes wielded more social power; (4) embracing a worldview dominated by simplistic binaries and intolerance; (5) widespread employment of conspiracy theories; (6) the labeling of truth and factual reporting as "fake news"; (7) the harnessing of the internet and social media to recruit, attack, and spread disinformation; and (8) suppression of opposing views. One by one, I started to see all of the facets of the online attacks against *Wuhan Diary* in China playing out on Twitter, Facebook, and the evening news in the United States; but instead of Fang Fang, the targets were people like Hunter Biden and Hillary Clinton; instead of Cyber Red Guards there were Proud Boys, conspiracy theories went by names like QAnon, and their mantra was Make America Great Again. Patterns of mutual reinforcement that we saw in the Chinese media between state media outlets, social media, and popular culture also appeared in the United States between baseless conspiracy theories about topics like election fraud mutually reinforced by online trolls, Fox News, and presidential tweets. And while government support of the Chinese trolls was somewhat ambiguous (perhaps the highest ranking government official to indirectly weigh in on the Fang Fang controversy was a tweet by Zhao Lijian), in the United States the president was openly retweeting conspiracy theories, expressing support for extremist groups, consistently spreading disinformation, and labeling media reports that did not align with his political views as "fake news." While Trump and his right-wing mob were China-bashing, Zhang Yiwu and the ultra-leftists in China were consistently attacking Trump. But the great irony is how these purported arch-enemies—the alt-right in the United States and the ultra-leftists in China—are actually perfect mirror images of one another, united in their jingoism, intolerance, and employment of social media to bully, intimidate, and threaten. In the words of Thomas Rid, "Disinformation operations, in essence, erode the very foundation of open societies—not only for the victim but also for the perpetrator."[20] For the United States, the pervasive spread of disinformation should be of particular concern, because it speaks to fissures in the health and stability of our very democracy. Again, quoting Rid, "The stronger and more robust a democratic body politic, the more resistant to disinformation it will be—and the more reluctant to deploy and optimize disinformation. Weakened democracies, in turn, succumb more easily to the temptations of active measures,"[21]

September 2020: I did a short interview with the *Los Angeles Times* about the controversy surrounding the Disney live-action remake of *Mulan*. When the article ran it included a short soundbite quote where I tried to contextualize the controversy surrounding the film. The following day I received a 2000-word email attack from an American reader in Santa Monica, California, who had taken offense to the quote. After having just spent the previous six months fending off online attacks and death threats on an almost daily basis, the irony was biting. A colleague from the UCLA medical school working on the front lines of the outbreak in Los Angeles treating COVID-19 patients was attacked by an online mob of right-wing pro-hydroxychloroquine trolls, and, a month later, one of my former doctoral advisees, now a professor at American University, gave an online lecture which was Zoom-bombed by people flashing white supremacist symbols and making threats of sexual violence … The trolls are indeed everywhere. The existential threats posed by online violence,

---

[20] Rid, Thomas. *Active Measures: The Secret History of Disinformation and Political Warfare*. New York: Farrar, Straus and Giroux, 2020. Pg. 11.
[21] Ibid.

disinformation campaigns, and extremist thought are just as real here as they are in China.

Lesson #4: Courage. When I first began to undertake the translation of Fang Fang's *Wuhan Diary*, I thought I was helping to give the author a voice, but what I discovered was that it was, in fact, she that had given me *my* voice. Most writers I know would have given in; under the threat of attacks and the constant political pressure, most writers would have stopped writing or caved in to pressure and not published the diary internationally. But Fang Fang pushed forward, knowing that history was on her side. The strength and resilience that Fang Fang demonstrated as she wrote *Wuhan Diary* and faced an unprecedented onslaught of online threats and attacks was one of the great acts of courage I have witnessed in my life. In particular, I remember shortly before publication as we were carrying out copyediting we were still waiting for Fang Fang to deliver her introduction. Given all of the scandals and attacks and the pressure to cancel publication, we were quite curious as to what her introduction would look like; I suspected she might adopt a more conciliatory tone to help ease the tensions. In her introduction, Fang Fang rhetorically asked why people have such a lax attitude during those first 20 days of the outbreak in Wuhan; she offered the following response:

> To be perfectly frank, part of the reason is that we had been too careless, and there are also objective life situations that contributed to that. But more important is the fact that we have placed too much faith in our government. We had faith that there was no way that the governmental leaders in Hubei Province would adopt such a lax and irresponsible attitude when it came to such a critical event where lives were in the balance. We also had faith that they would never hold fast to their "political correctness" and old ways of doing business in the face of a new threat that could affect the lives of millions of people. And we had faith that they would have better common sense and exercise better decision-making skills when a real threat was afoot. It was owing to that faith that I even sent a message to one of my WeChat groups saying: "The government would never dare to try to conceal something so huge." But in reality, as we now see how things have evolved, we know that a portion of the blame for this catastrophe lies with human error.
>
> Deeply ingrained habitual behaviors, like reporting the good news while hiding the bad, preventing people from speaking the truth, forbidding the public from understanding the true nature of events, and expressing a disdain for individual lives, have led to massive reprisals against our society, untold injuries against our people, and even terrible reprisals against those

officials themselves (a group of high-ranking Hubei officials have already been dismissed from office, while others who should bear additional responsibility still remain in office). All this, in turn, led to the city of Wuhan's falling under a 76-day quarantine, with its reverberations affecting untold numbers of people and places. It is absolutely essential that we continue to fight until those responsible are held accountable.[22]

As I read those words, a chill ran down my spine. Instead of the conciliatory tone I thought she might adopt, Fang Fang doubled down. For me it was not only a lesson in courage, but a lesson in dignity. A lesson about the importance of standing by your ideals, no matter what the cost, and never giving into the threats of bullies and trolls. Of course this book would not exist had it not been for *Wuhan Diary*, but I would have never had the fortitude and moral courage to write this book had it not been for Fang Fang's example. In the most unusual year of 2020, an era of division and lies, viral illness and viral attacks, the lesson of moral courage is perhaps the most essential. Fang Fang's diary presents not only a record of what occurred in Wuhan during the lockdown, but perhaps more importantly, a testament of the power of one woman's voice to resist one-dimensional hegemonic narratives and speak truth to power. In an online age of memes, soundbites, GIFs, and tweets, an age in which many have questioned the power of literature, Fang Fang's courage has shown us how a book can still galvanize a nation.

Then comes a **Lesson #5**, a lesson about **the Future**. 18 months after the initial Wuhan lockdown, detractors of Fang Fang's book in China claimed that *Wuhan Diary* missed its mark: for them, the failure of the West in controlling COVID-19 has accentuated China's success, rendering early mistakes (which Fang Fang highlighted in her diary) laughable as compared to the catastrophic losses suffered by countries like the United States. (Instead, nationalist Chinese trolls taunted me to write my own "American Diary" to document the high death toll and widespread infection rates in the United States.) Others view *Wuhan Diary* as a historical document, an explosive of-the-moment record of how a global crisis first unfolded, an eyewitness account that offered the world its first look at the damage this invisible virus was capable of unleashing and what a global lockdown might look like. It is this aspect of the "first look" which is

---

[22] Fang Fang. *Wuhan Diary: Dispatches from a Quarantined City*. New York: HarperVia, 2020. Pg. x–xi.

particularly important: while the entire world would eventually adjust to life under lockdown, there is no way to recapture the fear, trepidation, anger, and feelings of confusion, isolation, loss, and sadness that residents in Wuhan experienced during January and February of 2020. In this con text, Fang Fang's account provided a crucial archive of raw emotion, a record of responses, a museum of memories; it is this initial emotional response to COVID-19 which can never be reconstructed. In this sense, Fang Fang's account is a crucial touchstone for future readers to understand the affective dimensions of the early lockdown. But looking back, one of the most remarkable aspects of *Wuhan Diary* is just how prophetic the book would prove to be. 2020 was not just the year of COVID-19; it was also a year of discrimination and racial tension, disinformation campaigns, fake news, conspiracy theories, political division, and online violence. All of those keywords played a central role in Fang Fang's diary. It is in this context that *Wuhan Diary* offered the world not only a "first look" at the novel coronavirus, but also a "future look." Of course, there is an experiential symmetry in the ways that Fang Fang described experiences that seemed novel in January 2020—like wearing face masks, trying to reserve a delivery spot for online grocery deliveries, and the mundane aspects of life under quarantine, which she boiled down to "eating, sleeping, and binge watching"—however, on a much more profound level, Fang Fang was able to pinpoint the deeper fault lines extending out from behind the dark shadow of this virus.

Long before the racial reckoning of #BlackLivesMatter and #StopAsianHate, which swept over the United States against the backdrop of COVID-19, Fang Fang had already pinpointed the intersection of discrimination and the virus. The COVID-19 outbreak in the United States has been racialized on a number of different levels, from a sharp increase in instances of prejudice and hate crimes against Asian-Americans to the ways in which black, Hispanic, and indigenous communities were disproportionately afflicted with this virus. But even before the United States had a single documented case of the coronavirus, Fang Fang had already discussed the overt discrimination against Wuhan natives throughout China. Early on in the outbreak in China, one of the first responses to what was then broadly referred to in Chinese media as "Wuhan pneumonia" was widespread discrimination against Wuhan residents living, working, and traveling in other parts of China. It was a cogent warning of how rapidly disease unleashes paranoia, fear, discrimination, and an urge to isolate and "quarantine" racial, ethnic, and regional groups that are labeled as "infected." She also made it clear that the virus itself does not differentiate when it comes to race or class; as early as January 28, Fang Fang wrote "the virus doesn't discriminate between ordinary people and high-ranking leaders." At the very beginning of the COVID-19 pandemic, Fang Fang's diary offers all of us a glimpse not only of what was to come, but also how to face those challenges with grace, resolve, and courage. But most prophetic were Fang Fang's lessons on the issue of accountability.

Wuhan Diary also proved prescient in that the hate campaign used to suppress the book would become something of a playbook for future attempts to attack other public figures. One example can be seen in the hate campaign targeting film director Chloe Zhao in April 2021. Shortly after winning widespread accolades from Chinese state media after her film *Nomadland* won prizes at numerous top film festivals, an eight-year-old quote from an interview with *Filmmaker Magazine* where she allegedly described China as a place where "there are lies everywhere" was dredged up, resulting in a vicious online hate campaign and her film being barred from Chinese distribution. The parallels with the campaign against Fang Fang were evident: quotes were taken out of context and amplified; social media alit with a hate speech, which was later amplified by official state media; and ultimately works of the targeted individual were banned. A few months later in the fall of 2021, the pattern would repeat yet again—this time targeting Chinese-Canadian actor Simu Liu for comments he made during an interview in 2017 about his parents' reasons for immigrating to Canada. Again, the rather benign comments were amplified into a full-blown hate campaign and the commercial release of Liu's film *Shang-Chi* was blocked in China. Occurring at a crucial phase of tension between the United States and China, the campaign surrounding Fang Fang and the international publication of *Wuhan Diary* seemed to indeed set forth a pattern of how future cyber hate campaigns and disinformation campaigns would be developed. In almost all cases, small details (a description of abandoned cell phones, an old interview) are taken out of context and developed into an elaborate narrative that can be used to fan the flames of nationalist sentiment and targeted hatred (which are intertwined in that the offender is hated for "betraying" the nation) and used to achieve larger political or economic aims (banning a book that deviates from the "good story" or providing rationale for excluding Hollywood films from the Chinese market). With the increased frequency and tenacity of these online campaigns, learning how they function and evolve becomes an increasingly important lesson for the future.

Lesson #6: Accountability. This is a lesson that has not only transformed over time, but continues to be one of the most remarkable aspects of Fang Fang's *Wuhan Diary*. Fang Fang's repeated appeals for specialists and officials who mishandled the outbreak to stand up, take responsibility for their mistakes, and resign were a crucial part of the history of the early outbreak in Wuhan. At the same time, the stunning lack of accountability in countries all around the world would became a central facet of the COVID-19 pandemic and the ongoing ethical predicament. Fang Fang is referring to local officials who initially tried to cover up the severity of what was happening (including the silencing of the whistleblower Li Wenliang) and, in particular, takes aim at early assurances from health officials that person-to-person transmission of the coronavirus was not possible. As Fang Fang writes: "who were the leaders that in order to save face decided to twist the truth when reporting to their superiors and hide the truth from the public, who was it that put political correctness above the lives of our people, how many people contributed to this disaster? Whoever had a hand in this should take responsibility: the people need someone to assume accountability. At the same time, the government should urge officials from various departments whose actions misguided the public, leading to massive numbers of deaths, to resign."[23] Make no mistake, China did mishandle several key aspects of the novel coronavirus outbreak early on in Wuhan; however, they very quickly adopted a clear and strong policy that effectively flattened the curve and ultimately squashed the outbreak in China. As the United States gazed down the black hole of a dismantled pandemic response team; broken CDC test kits; chronic shortages of PPE and ventilators; delays in testing even when it was declared "anyone who wants a test can get a test"; a stunning lack of federal policy concerning COVID-19; a cesspool of lies, distraction, and disinformation; and a mounting death toll, we must ask who will hold *our* leaders accountable? If Fang Fang, writing under an authoritarian regime, under constant attack by thousands of internet trolls, was able to demand that her government live up to a higher standard of truth, transparency, and accountability, what is our excuse?

We should not forget that while Fang Fang and many Chinese citizens were deeply dissatisfied by a perceived lack of government accountability for early mistakes and the silencing of whistleblowers, the government *did*

---

[23] Fang Fang. *Wuhan Diary: Dispatches from a Quarantined City*. New York: HarperVia, 2020. Pg. 235–236.

dismiss numerous public officials from office based on their mishandling of the outbreak.[24] In mid-February Wuhan party secretary Ma Guoqiang 馬國強, Communist Party chief of the health commission of Hubei Zhang Jin 張晉, and Health Commission Director Liu Yingzi 劉英姿 were all fired or replaced; and in May Zhang Yuxin 張宇新, party secretary in charge of a residential complex in western Wuhan, was dismissed; and these are just a few of the Chinese officials who were purged in the wake of the outbreak. Were there others whose actions contributed to the health crisis that went unpunished? Perhaps. But what about the United States? With well over 990,000 deaths (as of April 2022) we witnessed a governmental failure on an unprecedented scale. And yet where are the public officials that have stood up to assume responsibility or been held accountable?

Two years after her diary went viral in China, Fang Fang's initial calls for accountability have been all but forgotten, buried under a smokescreen of attacks and threats against the author. Thanks to one of the most sophisticated and protracted personal attack campaigns waged against an individual, Fang Fang is now alternately referred to as "the witch of lies," a "traitor to China," a "secret CIA agent," and an entitled, out-of-touch *gongzhi* (a derogatory reference to "public intellectuals") who exploited the Chinese people to gain fame and profit. Here in the United States (and so many other Western nations that utterly failed when it came to the tests that COVID-19 presented to them), will this too be our "future look"? A long, dead, empty stare that, in the face of startling displays of inaction, ineptitude, and injustice, offers only silence, complacency, and cries of "victory" in our battle against the virus.

Finally, there is a lesson here about the nature of translation. Translation is an act of transmission. In the age of COVID-19 and, in the context of *Wuhan Diary*, transmission brings to mind multiple meanings: the transmission of the novel coronavirus, the transmission of Fang Fang's diary entries, and the transmission of the online attacks on the internet. For the trolls that attacked *Wuhan Diary*, translation was, in their eyes, an act of violence, an act of betrayal, an act of political aggression. According to one message a detractor of the book sent me: "Fang Fang's rotten stench will

---

[24] Fang Fang also acknowledges: "Several top officials in Hubei and Wuhan were removed from office" (xiii), in the preface to her diary.

last for 10,000 years and you will be the rag in which her corpse is wrapped." Is translation the dirty rag in which we bury the corpses of rotten ideas? Is it a weapon? Is it a virus? For the many netizens in China who have spent more than two years attacking *Wuhan Diary*, the answer to those questions is certainly an emphatic yes. While this goes against everything I have ever believed translation to be, I too must come to terms with the fact that just as readers can create meaning from texts that the author never intended, so too the *act of translation* itself can carry meaning never before intended by a translator. But translation can also speak to different forms of virality, a concept which has now emerged as one of the most important keywords of our post-COVID-19 era.

We are very much living in the age of virality: from online memes to presidential tweets and from conspiracy theories to deadly infections. While we often think of transmission in the case of disease or online attacks as forms of virality that corrupt us, weaken us, and leave us vulnerable to even more attacks, in the case of translation it can also build new layers of connective tissue between different cultures, bringing about understanding and communication where there was none. Derrida has written about the politics of hospitality as a continued test of sociality,[25] so too we can think of translation as a form of hospitality (and not hostility), a requisite act that invites "strangers" (readers of the target language) to engage in an experience that requires them to entertain and accommodate the ideas of the author. It is a process that not only expands our notions of civility, but also leaves valuable lessons for both the translator and the reader. For translation, at its heart is, of course, also an act of "transformation," that is, the rendering of one language into another. We rarely think of translation itself as a "transformative act," but that is precisely what it was to me. And so much of that transformation was a direct result of seeing the incredible model of strength and courage that Fang Fang presented. She inspired me to forge ahead and protect the truth, even if that sometimes meant making difficult choices. Part of that transformation involved a reevaluation of the ethics of translation itself. Throughout my career as a translator I have always seen my own invisibility as part of my professional responsibility. It is not about me; it is about the author's voice. Over the years, it has been a source of professional pride that the works I translate

---

[25] For more on the concept of hospitality, see: Derrida, Jacques. *Of Hospitality: Anne Dufourmantelle Invites Jacques Derrida to Respond.* Stanford: Stanford University Press, 2000.

do not bear *my* style, but the style the original work calls for in the target language. Though I found it deeply unsettling when the online trolls first attempted to draw ideological parallels between Fang Fang and myself, over the course of this protracted campaign, I have also emerged with new reflections on the role translation itself plays. The act of translating and reflecting upon *Wuhan Diary* has become an act of not only transmission, transformation, and hospitality, but also an act of activism and political engagement. That is something that I did not plan or anticipate when I began this journey; but thanks to Fang Fang's model (and, ironically, the attacks of thousands of online trolls), the invisible role of translation has been rendered visible, and, in the process, I have found my voice.

CHAPTER 12

Coda: The Light

In 2015 I contributed an article to a book entitled *A Journal of the Plague Year*, which was a catalogue exploring the 2003 SARS outbreak through the lens of literature, art, and film. My contribution was a chapter entitled "SARS@Hong Kong: A Brief Pathology of a Cinema of Disease." The article discusses a series of Hong Kong films from 2003 which explored the SARS outbreak against an earlier Hong Kong film from 1996 exploring the Ebola outbreak. While Herman Yau's 邱禮濤 *Ebola Syndrome* (*Yibola bingdu* 伊波拉病毒) was an unbridled work of exploitation cinema in which "disease is itself rendered 'abnormal,' 'perverted,' aligned with criminals, outcasts and the primitive,"[1] a later set of nearly a half dozen films about SARS expressed a vision that was conservative, comforting, and attempted to normalize disease within the context of the everyday. At the time, my argument was that when an actual outbreak occurs the possibilities for bold, experimental, and iconoclastic portrayals of disease dramatically retract. Instead, the 2003 SARS films showed us "the invention of a cinematic language to secularize and sterilize the SARS discourse through popular genres, group cinema forms, the power of celebrity, and an overriding nationalistic discourse. With the construction of this

---

[1] Berry, Michael. SARS@Hong Kong: A Brief Pathology of a Cinema of Disease. In *A Journal of the Plague Year*. Sternberg Press, 2015. Pg. 84.

M. Berry, *Translation, Disinformation, and Wuhan Diary*, https://doi.org/10.1007/978-3-031-16859-8_12

201

mini-genre, we simultaneously witness a narrowing of the generic conventions concerning how disease is narratized."[2]

Fast forward to early 2020, just as the outbreak in Wuhan was gaining attention worldwide, I had been commissioned to contribute an article to a journal in my field. Given the backdrop of the coronavirus outbreak, I thought my article on SARS and Hong Kong cinema from five years earlier might bear relevance to the current situation. The editor I had been communicating with loved the article, but the idea was eventually rejected by the editorial committee. The reason? The editorial board was concerned about the "humanitarian" angle: "Re-publishing an essay on SARS in [...] might be interpreted, especially by the Chinese readers, as an act of rubbing salt into the wound, and this is something [name of journal] does not want to be perceived as or accused of." I naturally respected the editorial board's decision; I was of course also aware of the uncertainties concerning the coronavirus outbreak and the potential for misunderstandings. At the same time, the journal's response inadvertently helped further validate the thesis of my original essay. That is, when an actual outbreak occurs, the ability to freely narratize disease becomes restricted. In this case, even this very observation proved too "sensitive" to discuss.

In some sense, this rather mundane editorial exchange (which was quickly resolved when I swapped out the SARS article for something else) would prove to be a warm-up exercise for much more powerful demonstration about how our ability to tell the story of an outbreak can become encumbered in unexpected and complex ways. When I wrote about SARS, it was clear that earlier works (like Herman's Yau's *Ebola Syndrome*), which took dramatic license with the presentation of disease, were no longer ethically permissible. But now with *Wuhan Diary* we witnessed something very different. Here was a diary rooted in fact and conveying the experience of witnessing, which also came under vicious attack. If radically creative and experimental narratives of disease are no longer permissible and truthful accounts like Fang Fang's are suppressed and attacked, then, one must ask, between truth and the imagination, what is left? Propagandistic cheerleading? Tear-jerking catharsis? Odes to victory?

After witnessing the brutal threats and attacks waged against Fang Fang and later experiencing firsthand what it feels like to be the target of a mass cyber trolling campaign, it is easy to become frustrated, disillusioned, and cynical. Having spent my entire adult life immersed in promoting Chinese

²Ibid. Pg. 99.

culture through education, programming, and publications, it was shattering to have my work misrepresented and attacked and my integrity called into question. And it was equally devastating to stand by and see Fang Fang's work being systematically discredited and written off as lies. But as the online attacks raged, there were also signs of a true civil society that began to shine through from behind the cracks in the trolls' wall of anger and malice.

Following the initial flood of attacks, there were those that dared to directly challenge the trolls on Weibo. They would point out the absurdity with short jabs like:

> It looks like you have been a Red Guard so long that now you can't stand the fact that you cannot immigrate to North Korea.
> Everyone posting on this message board have all gone insane!
> I'm shocked by these comments…At the end of the day, are these the voices that represent us? Voices of ignorance and spite? This younger generation is terrifying
> It is, after all, just a book; what is there for all these Chinese people to be so terrified about? And they are even threatening the writer? Threatening the translator? I really don't get it….is it really the author that is "passing the knife" [to the West] or is it this group of Red Assassins passing the knife?

Public voices of support were still largely outnumbered by the trolls, but they were there in the message threads, tucked in between the death threats and slanderous accusations. Many of them commented on how the message board felt like a time machine taking them back to 1968; for many it indeed felt like a digital Cultural Revolution.

Friends who learned of the attacks began to send me texts and emails to express their support; famous Chinese writers and filmmakers that I never met also reached out. One award-winning novelist whose work I had admired for nearly 20 years tracked down my email and sent an incredibly moving letter of support.

> Friends in China told me about the brutal verbal attacks on you for undertaking the task of translating and managing the publication of Fang Fang's Wuhan diary. Such irrational behavior reminds me only too closely of the horror of the Cultural Revolution, of which I feel deeply ashamed. This letter is to let you know that, while fully respecting freedom of speech, I and my friends […] do not condone such behavior. Your lifelong dedication to the cause of introducing Chinese literature to the world is deeply appreciated by many of us, and the flying dust may obscure the view of some, but definitely not all.

There were also many friends who reached out but didn't once mention the attacks or Fang Fang—they know that doing so could be construed as moving into "sensitive" terrain—instead they simply sent short texts inviting me to dinner next time I'm in Beijing or simply wishing me well. But their intentions were clear and their gestures were appreciated. Likely due to the threat of reprisals, most of those messages came as private messages, emails, and texts. Then on April 16, 2020, an article entitled "Professor Michael Berry" began widely circulating on Weibo.

The article was written by Zhang Sheng 張生, a Chinese literature professor at Tongji University in Shanghai who is also an acclaimed novelist. Nearly a decade earlier, while I was still teaching at UCSB, I had hosted Zhang Sheng as a visiting scholar. It was a somewhat tumultuous time in my life; my son was a year old and I had just begun to develop a serious autoimmune disorder which would go undiagnosed for more than a year. I always regretted that I was unable to spend more time with Professor Zhang, but nevertheless treasured our many long conversations while he was in Santa Barbara. It had been several years since we were in touch and the appearance of the essay caught me off guard. The essay did not once mention the words "Fang Fang" or "Wuhan Diary," nor did it discuss the US-China trade war, COVID-19, or any of the other trending topics of the day. Instead Zhang Sheng's long essay offered a touching first-person portrait of me as a scholar and human being and chronicle of our friendship. Just in case readers didn't get the intention behind this gesture, Zhang Sheng concluded his essay thus:

> I've always been fond of something the scholar Hu Shi 胡適 once said: "To stand up for those who have been unjustly slandered is the first principle of justice." Seeing this group of people using such dirty language and malicious intentions to hurt a professor who has so passionately supported Chinese literature and film, I feel a need to speak out; at the same time, I hope these words are able to provide Michael with a bit of warmth and consolation; I don't want him to think that I am just yet another member of the silent crowd of onlookers.[3]

I'm sure that Zhang Sheng knew that by stepping into the muddy waters of a heated online attack campaign, he was opening himself up to also be

[3] Zhang Sheng 張生. "Professor Michael Berry" ("Bai Ruiwen jiaoshou" 白睿文教授) originally posted to Weibo on April 16, 2020, reprinted on numerous websites, including: https://posts.careerengine.us/p/5ead539fff7e81298ce3071a.

targeted by personal attacks. He did it anyway. It was the kind of gesture that under normal circumstances one would not consider extraordinary, but in the context of that moment, given the rising tensions between the United States and China and deep social fissures tearing through society, it became an act of great courage. In some sense, that is also the story of *Wuhan Diary*. There shouldn't be anything extraordinary about publishing an online diary but the circumstances surrounding its politicization and attacks transformed Fang Fang's actions into a rare act of social engagement and defiance.

After the first few days of attacks around April 9 and 10, I decided to take a short break from Weibo, even temporarily shutting down the message boards on my posts. But roughly a week later, around the time Zhang Sheng posted his essay, I opened the private message box on my Weibo app to discover my inbox filled with new messages. My heart dropped, assuming they contained more attacks and death threats. There were a few, but instead I found something else.

Hundreds upon hundreds of messages filled with support, love, and hope. Between May 12 and May 16 I received approximately 2000 messages. Many were just short notes of apology or expressions of support. The individuals writing used a mixture of Chinese, English, and sometimes just emojis, like the person who just sent me rows of hearts and flowers. And then there were others who expressed their support in other ways, such as a user who sent me a series of pictures: five images of adorable baby kittens and bunnies. I got the message. But many of them expressed something much deeper, revealing more profound insights into Chinese society. Where did these messages come from? Around the same time that Zhang Sheng published his public defense of my character, Fang Fang had also begun to come out to publicly correct the lies and slanderous statements that had been circulating about me. She did so through Weibo (where she has over four million followers) and through interviews with official media outlets where she attempted to directly challenge the twisted conspiracy theories being endorsed by the ultra-nationalist trolls. I believe those letters came from Fang Fang's supporters who had been following the online persecution campaign and felt they needed to speak out.

After months of non-stop media coverage about the online attacks and online persecution that Fang Fang and, to a much lesser extent, I have received, it is important to preserve the other side of the story. Unlike the attacks, which appear in headline articles and public messages, these words of support came in the form of private messages. Many of these users know that posting in public runs the risk of opening themselves up to troll attacks, so these supporters are forced to remain largely invisible. While I have not posted the users' names in order to protect their identities, their voices are no longer silent. They represent the true "silent majority" in China—decent fair-minded people who are often unable to openly express their true sentiments about "sensitive" topics, even if it just one woman's diary. The trolls carry big sticks and make a lot of noise, but these are the voices that represent the true conscience of the nation and it is to them I give the final word:

> I'm not sure if you are still reading your Weibo messages, but if you are, I hope you won't be shocked by all of the malicious messages that have been flooding your profile. There are a lot of us out there that believe Fang Fang had no ill intent in deciding to publish her diary abroad.
>
> I felt terribly sorry when I saw the internet violence you were subjected to for translating Fang Fang's *Wuhan Diary*. Please don't pay any attention to all of these rumors and malicious comments. Nationalist sentiments are currently extremely high in China today and it has already gotten to the point where diverse voices are barely tolerated. One day, future generations will look back upon these curses and attacks and laugh at them. Wishing you all the best!
>
> Hi Michael, I'm an interpreter/translator. Sorry to see that you got verbally bullied just because you translated someone's diary. I have no comment on Fang Fang's work but I think it's unfair to ask the translator to be held accountable for the authenticity of the content. And people assume you pick side just because you translate something. It's a joke. Most of the time, they find translators/interpreters as the scapegoat of disagreements, but this time, sadly, you are their target, which is irrational, unjustified and nonsense. Well, I don't know what else I can say, take care.
>
> Hi Michael, I know it'll be hard to disregard all these ridiculous and insulting comments, but please know that there are sensible people still left and these clowns aren't representations of everyone. I loved your books and they helped in my own study of filmmaking. You are appreciated! And I believe you'll do the translation justice!!! So sorry about this madness going on. I wish it would all stop.
>
> Please don't take those Weibo comments to heart, they represent the very worst side of Chinese netizens. Recently the evil tendencies on Weibo are getting worse and worse; as a normal Chinese citizen I was absolutely shocked by what I read in the comments section of your account; those attacks left me quite depressed, I feel like I almost have PTSD after reading those attacks. [crying emoji]

Hi Mr. Berry, it's a shame that so many people leave racial or nationalism comments under your posts. Statistics show that most of the Weibo users haven't finished high school. Whatever, keep happy and healthy.

I just want to say I support you. Just ignore those flies.

Hi, How are you? Now I am sending this message to you to thank you for translating Ms Fang Fang's diary. It is a shame that the guidance of public opinion in China is terrible, but please believe that there are still many people who support Ms. Fang Fang and thank you very much for your hard working! My hometown is Wuhan so I know exactly what happened in this city. History will remember Fang Fang and all the brave people. Take care and best wishes.

Mr. Berry please pay no heed to those ignorant comments.

Justice lies within our hearts.

Freedom will provide the final judgement of what is right and wrong.

Pay no heed to those who attempt to slander you with malicious comments.

They are only using you and Fang Fang to release their frustrations.

They are but a mob of the mindless.

Reading the comments on your Weibo page has been a painful experience for me. Please don't lose hope in the youth of China. Within China today discourse has turned to extremist positions; those irrational post are encouraged while more rational people are forced to shut up; but we are still finding ways to express ourselves and encourage those around us to stay reasonable and maintain civility. I wish you and your family health and happiness. I was born in 1995 and went to college here in China; I too am a student. I would like to express my support and appreciation for your hard work in trying to bring Eastern and Western culture closer together. Reading through some of the recent posts on your account there are nearly 4,000 messages and most are overwhelming expressions of support for you. You can see that rational and reasonable people are the majority.

Dear sir: Literature is beautiful, as is the Chinese language. But today even I as a Chinese person feel deeply disappointed in the Chinese internet. [three crying emojis] Please don't read Weibo anymore, there is simply too much racism and prejudice here. When they use the beautiful Chinese language to attack and insult you, I feel such profound sadness and hopelessness. And so I send you a line of poetry from Bei Dao, who just yesterday was also a victim of online violence. [crying emoji] "You didn't return when you said you were coming, and this is the meaning of departure." Finally, I want to wish you peace and happiness in your everyday life; I hope your country can quickly emerge from the shadow of COVID-19.

I was utterly shocked to see the comments posted on your Weibo account. Thank you for translating Fang Fang's diary. I hope you don't take the attacks by those Little Pinks to heart. Actually, I hope those posts become first-hand research material to express the ideological divide and extremism present in Chinese society today.

Dear Prof, please ignore the comment in your Weibo. I can't represent them but I personally apologize for their ignorance and racism. They are just a small part of Chinese people, chess of the politicians, manipulated by propaganda. They don't really understand what they're doing. There are many people like me who're shamed of them…

Professor Berry: Please ignore the ill-will contained in those comments; I feel ashamed that there are people who are so rude and irrational. Political ideology has made them crazy.

No matter what the original work says, it is not the fault of the translator.

I'm so sorry. This country has gone mad. There's nothing I can do.

Don't feel bad for those comments, they should be normal people, but I guess you know the new China's new education is very red, they just in difficult time and be brain washed. (sic)

I would like to express my apologies. We are caught in an era of deep division; they are the minority. I hope you aren't negatively impacted by them. Please keep doing what you do; it is difficult, but it is the right thing to do. Finally, thank you for supporting Chinese culture.

As a Chinese, I apologize for the insults and defamation of thse Chinese ultra-leftists who we call "XiaoFenHong" (Little Pinks) or the Nazis. These people only represent a part of the Chinese who have not received a good education…Thank you for the Wuhan Diary and for promoting the democratization of Chinese society.

[…] Although I personally feel that there was indeed some issues concerning oversight with the original online introduction of Fang Fang's diary in English, which was somewhat skewed, I still feel that the diary deserves to be published if the translation is accurate. I hope that on some level this book will help bridge the gap between the prejudices running through the East and the West. I learned that the comments section on your Weibo page had fallen under attack by the so-called "keyboard avengers," I feel the despicable language and ignorance of this relatively small subset of society is shameful. Actually, I feel that the entire world has entered a new low point, don't you? I hope you are not impacted by those radical attacks; perhaps they will offer you a brand new understanding of China as it goes through a period of radical transformation. As the coronavirus unleashes its havoc, I hope you and your family will remain safe and healthy.

Hello, I just saw the comments on your Weibo page and, as a Chinese, I feel such deep shame, embarrassment, anger, and helplessness. There is so little I can do…but as I am unable to change the deeply entrenched prejudices of others, I commit to be the best I can be. I commit to stick to my ideals and not be contaminated by the dirty flood around me, never act in collusion with them or take the side of the evildoers. Here I would like to apologize to you on behalf of those who have insulted you. I also want to thank you for translating Fang Fang's diary into English, let the entire world witness what occurred at the epicenter…

Not all Chinese people are like this, please believe me. If you have the opportunity to explain this extreme behavior of patriots on Twitter, please also tell netizens around the world that there are also people who pursue individualism and liberalism in China, but I am sorry that we have not done enough, we are still under the control of the government because, in contrast, the comments of the ultra-patriots are more popular than those of the individualists and liberals. Even so, citizens who pursue liberalism and individualism in China have the same heart as citizens who are pursuing individualism and liberalism worldwide.

We will still fight, though the road is full of uncertainty. But we will never give up the pursuit of freedom, nor will we kill the opportunity to pursue freedom by the acts of extreme patriots.

Some time ago, some Chinese extreme patriots and Thai netizens said, this phenomenon is the same as your message below Weibo.

Because of uninformable reasons, China cannot tweeted. This has caused many netizens around the world to misunderstand Chinese netizens. Because to a great extent, the patriots have a lot of remarks, they are organized and premeditated. Because if there is an extreme patriot, there will be countless extreme patriots. This is like Pandora's magic box, which cannot be closed when opened. Their remarks sometimes represent individualist remarks.

But as liberals, we don't want to be represented by the patriots' remarks. At the same time, our hearts are also connected with our compatriots in Hong Kong and Taiwan. We respect their ideas and hope they are happy. Sometimes it is precisely because of them that they bring hope to those who are pursuing individualism and liberalism in mainland China. We are very grateful to them.

I feel deep shame about the way netizens have been speaking about you in online posts. There is a deep fissure in online culture, especially during an unusual time like this. The road to enlightenment is long…as is the road to civility. Chinese culture is still on that road and moments of hope and hopelessness are inevitable along the way, but neither of us are standing on the sidelines.

BIBLIOGRAPHY

Anonymous. "Some Chinese intellectuals hold distorted values, represented by Fang Fang: academician Zhang Boli" The Global Times. May 14, 2020a. https://www.globaltimes.cn/content/1188347.shtml

Anonymous. "Lei Lei Wants to Beat "Failed" Woman Writer While Xu Xiaodong Calls on the Martial World to Protect Fang Fang (雷雷要凑败家女作家 徐晓冬 吁武林:保护方方) Published on aboluowang 阿波羅新聞 April 17, 2020b. https://www.aboluowang.com/2020/0417/1438226.html

Bandurski, David. "PLA Site Attacks Bad Domestic Media" China Media Project, June 23, 2020. https://chinamediaproject.org/2020/06/23/caixin-online-called-anti-china-over-fang-fang-diary-publication/

Bao, Hongwei. "Three Woman and Their Wuhan Diaries: Women's Writing in a Quarantined Chinese City" Cha Journal. October 17, 2020. https://chajournal.blog/2020/10/17/wuhan-diaries/?fbclid=IwAR0Nj1WeJMcfA1ewUI729bIO9PQy74vO7pX1W_dcAM_BooJ0gTcpk91GoBI

Becker, Jasper. *Made in China: Wuhan, COVID and the Quest for Biotech Supremacy*. London: C. Hurst & Co. 2021.

Bengali, Shashank and Alice Su. "'Put on a mask and shut up': China's new 'Wolf Warriors' spread hoaxes and attack a world of critics" Los Angeles Times. May 4. 2020. https://www.latimes.com/world-nation/story/2020-05-04/wolf-warrior-diplomats-defend-china-handling-coronavirus

Berry, Michael. *A History of Pain: Trauma in Modern Chinese Literature and Film*. New York: Columbia University Press.

Berry, Michael. SARS@Hong Kong: A Brief Pathology of a Cinema of Disease. In *A Journal of the Plague Year*. Sternberg Press, 2015.

© The Author(s), under exclusive license to Springer Nature Switzerland AG 2022
M. Berry, *Translation, Disinformation, and Wuhan Diary*,
https://doi.org/10.1007/978-3-031-16859-8

211

Blanchette, Jude D.. *China's New Red Guards: The Return of Radicalism and the Rebirth of Mao Zedong.* New York: Oxford University Press, 2019.

Bondes, Maria and Gunter Schucher, "Derailed emotions: The transformation of claims and targets during the Wenzhou online incident" in Wenhong Chen (ed.) *The Internet, Social Networks and Civic Engagement in Chinese Societies.* Routledge, 2015.

Carter, Liz. *Let 100 Voices Speak: How the Internet is Transforming China and Changing Everything.* New York: I.B. Tauris, 2015.

Chang Liu. "Chinese Young Nationalists amid The COVID-19 Pandemic: A Rap against A "Diary" online essay published on the New School Transregional Center for Democratic Studies," July 20, 2020. https://blogs.newschool. edu/tcds/2020/07/20/chinese-young-nationalists-amid-the-covid-19-pandemic-a-rap-against-a-diary/

Chen, Kaiping, Anfan Chen, Jingwen Zhang, Jingbo Meng, and Cuihua Shen. "Conspiracy and debunking narratives about COVID-19 origins on Chinese social media: How it started and who is to blame" *Misinformation Review.* December 10, 2020a. https://misinforeview.hks.harvard.edu/article/conspiracy-and-debunking-narratives-about-covid-19-origins-on-chinese-social-media-how-it-started-and-who-is-to-blame/

Chen Liansong 陳聯松 and Zhao Wenying 趙文穎. The Doctor's Pandemic Diary: COVID 19 in 2020 (Yiqing zaji: Yigashidai de chuangkou 疫情雜記:一個時代的窗口). California, Qiao Publishing, 2020.

Chen Xi. "'Wuhan Girl A Nian Diary' – young Chinese woman's tough experience during COVID-19 lockdown moves readers" November 6, 2020. *The Global Times.* https://www.globaltimes.cn/content/1205924.shtml

Chen, Xinyu., Zhuo, Zenghua., Xu, Yichen. and Wu, Zhihang. (2020b), Report of a Survey on Fang Fang Diary ('Fang Fang Riji Wenjuan Diaocha Yanjiu Baogao' 方方日記問卷調查研究報告), China Law Review (Zhongguo Falu Pinglun 中國法律評論), available at: https://wemp.app/posts/299b0cb7-4 1b3-4c5b-9f32-e06e145ac9ca.

Cui Yongyuan 崔永元. "A Lesson for Fang Fang" (Gei Fang Fang shang yi ke 給方方生一課). https://www.xiaxiaoqiang.net/previous-lesson/.html

Chen, Wenhong (ed.). *The Internet, Social Networks and Civic Engagement in Chinese Societies.* Routledge, 2015.

Dai Qing 戴晴. *Wang Shiwei and Wild Lilies: Rectification and Purges in the Chinese Communist Party 1942–1944.* Routledge, 1993.

David, Deborah and Helen Siu (eds.). *SARS: Reception and Interpretation in three Chinese Cities.* Routledge, 2007.

Davidson, H. "Chinese writer faces online backlash over Wuhan lockdown diary." The Guardian, April 10, 2020. https://www.theguardian.com/world/2020/apr/10/chinese-writer-fang-fang-faces-online-backlashwuhan-lockdown-diary

Derrida, Jacques. *Of Hospitality: Anne Dufourmantelle Invites Jacques Derrida to Respond*. Stanford: Stanford University Press, 2000.

Fang Fang 方方. *Wuhan Diary: Dispatches from a Quarantined City*. Translated by Michael Berry. New York: HarperVia, 2020.

Fang Fang 方方. "About: Exploiting Misery" ("Guanyu: Maican" 關於:賣慘) originally published on WeChat and reposted on Radio France International, n.d. https://www.rfi.fr/cn/中国/20200505-方方-关于-5-关于卖惨

Fang Fang 方方 *Selected Works of Fang Fang* (*Fang Fang zixuanji* 方方自選集). Beijing: Tiandi Press, 2018.

Fang Fang 方方. *A Soft Burial* (*Ruan mai* 軟埋). Beijing: Renmin Publishing House, 2016.

Fedtke, Jana, Mohammed Ibahrine, and Yuting Wang. "Corona crisis chronicle: Fang Fang's *Wuhan Diary* (2020) as an act of sousveillance" *Online Information Review* February 23, 2021. https://www.emerald.com/insight/1468-4527.htm

Feng Chuan 馮川. *Criticism of Fang Fang's Diary* (*Fang Fang riji pipan* 方方日記批判) e-book, 2020. No publisher listed. Reprinted on line at Wuyou zhi xiang wangkan 烏有之鄉網刊 under the alternate title *Text, Logic, and Problems with Fang Fang's Diary* (*Fang Fang riji de wenben, luojiyuwenti* 《方方日記》的文本、邏輯與問題) http://www.wyzxwk.com/Article/yulun/2020/05/417613.html)

Feng, Yang. *A New Virus: The start of the pandemic*. Yang Feng, 2020.

Gao, Xibai (ed.). *China's Novel Coronavirus Response: Guidelines for Governments, Communities, Entities and Individuals to Combat COVID-19*. Lisa Cella Press, 2020.

Garner, Dwight. "'Wuhan Diary' offers an angry and eerie view from inside quarantine." New York Times, May 21, 2020. https://www.pilotonline.com/entertainment/books/vp-db-book-wuhan-diary-fang-fang-review-052420-20200521-jqliwdybibhl7ph4m7aa4sowye-story.html

Gladstone, Rick. "Trump Demands U.N. Hold China to Account for Coronavirus Pandemic" New York Times, Dept. 22, 2020. https://www.nytimes.com/2020/09/22/world/americas/UN-Trump-Xi-China-coronavirus.html

Griffiths, James. *The Great Firewall of China: How to Build and Control an Alternative Version of the Internet*. London: Zed Books, 2019.

Grogan, Bryan. "Chinese Rapper's Diss Track Aims at Austrian Prime Minister Scott Morrison" in RADII, December 6, 2020. https://radiichina.com/bo-peep-scott-morrison/

Guo Jing 郭晶. *Diary of the Wuhan Lockdown* (*Wuhan fengcheng riji* 武漢封城日記). Taipei: Linking, 2020.

Hernandez, Javier C. "As China Cracks Down on Coronavirus Coverage, Journalists Fight back" New York Times, March 14, 2020. https://www.nytimes.com/2020/03/14/business/media/coronavirus-china-journalists.html

Hu Xijin 胡錫進. "Huxijin's Take on the "Fang Fang Diary" Phenomena" ("Hu Xijin ping 'Fang Fang riji' xianxiang" 胡錫進評方方日記現象) Global Times 環球時報, March 19, 2020. https://news.ifeng.com/c/7uyH0zY3rsm

Jing Wu, Simin Li, and Hongzhe Wang. "From Fans to "Little Pink" in Hailong Liu ed. *From Cyber-Nationalism to Fandom Nationalism: The Case of Diba Expedition in China.* New York: Routledge, 2020.

Kewalramani, Manoj. *Smokeless War: China's Quest for Geopolitical Dominance.* New Delhi: Bloomsbury India, 2021.

Kraidy, Marwan M.. *The naked Blogger of Cairo: Creative Insurgency in the Arab World.* Cambridge, Harvard University Press, 2016.

Lai Fu 來福. "The Battle Over Fang Fang: Old Answers and New Questions to the 'Theory of Passing the Knife'" (Fang Fang Zhanzheng: Tidaolun dejiuda'an he xin wenti方方戰爭:「剃刀論」的舊答案和新問題) Initium Media, May 20, 2020. https://theinitium.com/article/20200515-opinion-fangfang-people-war-national-socialism/

Lao Yang Daochushuo 老楊到處說. "Is Fang Fang a Member of the Freemasons!?" ("Fang Fang shi Gongjihuiyuan!?" 方方是共濟會員!?) posted to Youtube on December 2, 2020: https://www.youtube.com/watch?v=usc8wShVEuw

Lee, Claire Seunggeun. *Soft Power: Made in China.* Palgrave Macmillan, 2018.

Lei Lei 雷雷. n.d. "Founder of Thunder God Tai Chi Lei Lei Challenges Fang Fang" (雷公太极创始人雷雷挑战方方) was uploaded to various social media platforms and widely disseminated online, including the following website: https://www.wenxuecity.com/news/2020/04/21/9383521.html

Levine, Suzanne Jill. *The Subversive Scribe: Translating Latin American Fiction.* Dalkey Archive, 2009.

Li, Jie and Enhua Zhang (eds.). *Red Legacies in China: Cultural Afterlives of the Cultural Revolution.* Harvard University Asia Center, 2016.

Li Jing 黎靖 (written and illustrated). *2020 Wuhan Diary* (2020 *Wuhan riji* 2020 武漢日記). Beijing: Zhongguo guojiguangbo chubanshe, 2020.

Liao Guangsheng 廖光生. *Exclusionism and Chinese Politics* (*Paiwai yu Zhongguo zhengzhi* 排外與中國政治). Taipei: Sanmin shuju, 1986. Pg. 136.

Liu, Hailong ed. *From Cyber-Nationalism to Fandom Nationalism: The Case of Diba Expedition in China.* New York: Routledge, 2020.

Liu Yu 劉宇. *I'm Afraid I Might One Day Forget: A Record of Fighting the Outbreak in Wuhan* (*Wo pa jianglai hui wangji: Wuhan kangyi shouji* 我怕將來會忘記:武漢抗疫手記). Hong Kong: Joint Publishing, 2020.

Lu Guoping 魯國平先生. "Are we being too hard on Fang Fang by criticizing her diary as a work of 'hearsay'?" ("Zhize fangfang riji daotingtushuo shi keqiu ma" 指責方方日記"道聽途說"是苛求嗎?) Sina.com, April, 23, 2020. https://k.sina.cn/article_1142648704_441b6f8001900m7a6.html

Lu, Pinyue. (2020) "Fang Fang's Diary: An Indefensible Mistake, International Critical Thought" in *International Political Thought* Volume 10, 2020, Issue 3 pg. 483–493. DOI: https://doi.org/10.1080/21598282.2020.1823612

Luo Siling 羅四鴒. "After Being Attacked by Leftists, Fang Fang Discussed the 'Soft Burial' of *Soft* Burial" (Zaodao zuopai weigong zuojia Fang Fang tan ruanmai de ruanmai" 遭左派圍攻，作家方方談《軟埋》的"軟埋") in The New York Times Chinese Edition. June 27, 2017. https://cn.nytimes.com/china/20170627/cc27fang-fang/

Lu Hsun. *Selected Stories*. New York: W.W. Norton, 2003.

McDougall, Bonnie S.. *Mao Zedong's "Talks at the Yan'an Conference on Literature and Art: A Translation of the 1943 Text with Commentary.*" University of Michigan, Center for Chinese Studies, 1980.

McGregor, Richard. *Xi Jinping: The Backlash*. Penguin Books, 2019.

Mengin, Francoise (ed.). *Cyber China: Reshaping National Identities in the Age of Information*. Palgrave Macmillan, 2004.

Min Jiang and Ashley Esaray, "Uncivil Society in Digital Society: Incivility, Fragmentation, and Political Stability" in *International Journal of Communication*. Vol 12 (2018). https://ijoc.org/index.php/ijoc/article/view/9478/2340

Miyajima, Kanako. "Author of 'Wuhan Diary' now finds herself muzzled in China" The Asahi Shimbun, December 15, 2020. http://www.asahi.com/ajw/articles/13988776

Ng, Jason Q.. *Blocked on Weibo*. New York, The New Press, 2013.

Ni Ke 尼克. *Going Home: A Record of Taiwanese Stranded in Wuhan and Their Escape from a Quarantined City* (*Fanjia: Hubei Wuhan shoukun taiwanren fengcheng taoyiji* 返家:湖北武漢受困台灣人封城逃疫記). Taipei: China Times, 2020.

Perper, Rosie. "A 4th Chinese citizen journalist was reportedly detained while livestreaming what life was like in Wuhan at the height of the coronavirus outbreak." May 18, 2020 Business Insider. https://www.businessinsider.com/zhang-zhan-fourth-chinese-journalist-arrested-for-livestreaming-in-wuhan-2020-5

Pottinger, Matthew. "Remarks by Deputy National Security Advisor Matt Pottinger to the Miller Center at the University of Virginia" are available in text format here: https://www.whitehouse.gov/briefings-statements/remarks-deputy-national-security-advisor-matt-pottinger-miller-center-university-virginia/ or in video format here: https://www.youtube.com/watch?v=dp5h6n6fbUg

Rao Yufeng 饒玉峰 and Huang Yuqi 黃昱綺. "The Lightspeed Publication of 'Fang Fang's Diary' Will Only Expose the Truth About More Western 'Pot Throwing.'" ("Guangshu chubande FangFang riji, zhineng baolu gengduo xifang 'shuaiguo' de zhenxiang" 光速出版的《方方日記》，只能暴露更多西方"甩鍋"的真相)

June 10, 2020 on China Military (Zhongguo junwang 中國軍網): http://
www.81.cn/jwgd/2020-06/10/content_9832032.htm

Renmin wang 人民網. *The People's Battle Against COVID-19* (*Renmin zhanyi* 人
民戰疫). Chongqing: Chongqing chubanshe, 2020.

Roberts, Margaret E. *Censored: Distraction and Diversion Inside China's Great
Firewall.* Princeton: Princeton University Press, 2018a.

Robins, Kevin. "The Great City is Fragile: Fang Fang's *Wuhan Diary.*" *Cultural
Politics,* Volume 17, Issue 1. Duke University Press, 2021.

Rojas, Carlos. *Homesickness: Culture, Contagion, and National Transformation in
Modern China.* Cambridge: Harvard University Press, 2015a.

Rid, Thomas. *Active Measures: The Secret History of Disinformation and Political
Warfare.* New York: Farrar, Straus and Giroux, 2020.

Roberts, Margaret E.. *Censored: Distraction and Diversion Inside China's Great
Firewall.* Princeton: Princeton University Press, 2018b.

Rojas, Carlos. *Homesickness: Culture, Contagion, and National Transformation in
Modern China.* Cambridge: Harvard University Press, 2015b.

Sayed, Adham (Adeham Saiyide 阿德漢 賽義德). *Confidence Comes from
Effectiveness: A Foreigner's Wuhan Diary* (*Jianding: Yige waiguoren de Wuhan
riji* 堅定:一個外國人的武漢日記). Beijing: The Contemporary World
Press, 2020.

Sima Nan 司馬南. "Critique of Fang Fang Being Awarded the Emile Guimet Prize
for Asian Literature" (Sima Nan: Ping Fang Fang you huo Faguo Jimei wenxuejiang 司馬南:評方方又獲吉美文學獎) Youtube video uploaded on January
28, 2021. https://www.youtube.com/watch?v=dnrqtRXTPRg

Sina Weibo, Sina Reading 新浪微博. *Wuhan Diary of Resistance Against the Virus*
(*Wuhan kangyi riji* 武漢抗疫日記). Beijing: Beijing lianhe chubanshe, 2020.

Sinha, Mrinalini. *Specters of Mother India: The Global Restructuring of an Empire.*
Durham: Duke University Press, 2006.

Subramani, A. "ICJ moves UNHRC against China for COVID-19 reparations"
April 2, 2020 Times of India. https://timesofindia.indiatimes.com/india/icj-
moves-unhcr-against-china-for-covid-19-reparations/articleshow/7496
5784.cms

Tietouwa 鐵頭娃. "Publication date of the English edition of Fang Fang's Diary
has been moved up, becoming a true bullet." ("Fang Fang yingwenban riji tiqian chuban, zhen chengle yike zidan" 方方英文版日記提前出版, 真誠了一顆
子彈),May 2, 2020. https://dy.163.com/article/FBK3GTEQ053717V3.html

Tooze, Adam. *Shutdown: How Covid Shook the World's Economy.* New York:
Viking, 2021.

Various authors. *Stories of Courage and Determination: Wuhan in Coronavirus
Lockdown.* Beijing: Foreign Language Press, 2020a.

Various authors. *Yazhou Zhoukan: The International Chinese Newsweekly* April
20–26, 2020b issue. Special issue on *Wuhan Diary.*

Various authors. *INK Literary Monthly*. May 2020c. Special issue on Coronavirus disease of 2019.

Veg, Sebastian. *Minjian: The Rise of China's Grassroots Intellectuals*. New York, Columbia University Press, 2019.

"Voice of the Dragon" (Long zhi sheng 龍之聲) "Headline News Today! They Have Dug Out the Dirt! There is a Huge Secret Lurking Within Fang Fang's Villa That No One Can Imagine! The Socking Scandal is Now Exposed for All to See!" ("Jinri toutiao! Zhongyu chachulai le! Fang Fang bieshu laowu ancang yizhuang jingtian da mimi, chaochu le suoyouren xiangxiang! Jingtianheimu baoguang, dabaiyutianxia!" 今日頭條!終於查出來了!方方別墅老屋暗藏一樁驚天動地的秘密，超出了所有人想像!驚天黑幕爆光大白於天下!) Youtube video uploaded on April 29, 2020: https://www.youtube.com/watch?v=87EKrim11DI

Walsh, Joe. "Trump if Demanding China Pay 'Big Price' for Covid-19" October 8, 2020. Forbes. https://www.forbes.com/sites/joewalsh/2020/10/08/trump-is-demanding-china-pay-big-price-for-covid-19/#1faf5c5841c8

Wang, David Der-wei. *Why Fiction Matters in Contemporary China*. Waltham, MA: Brandeis University Press, 2020.

Wang, Tuo. *The Cultural Revolution and Overacting: Dynamics Between Politics and Performance*. Lanham: Lexington Books, 2014.

Wang, Vivian and Javier C. Hernandez. "China Long Avoided Discussing Mental Health. The Pandemic Changed That." New York Times, December 21, 2020. https://www.nytimes.com/2020/12/21/world/asia/china-covid-mental-health.html

Wang, Zheng. *Never Forget National Humiliation: Historical Memory in Chinese Politics and Foreign Relations*. New York: Columbia University Press, 2012.

Wu Rui 吳銳. Twentieth Century Chinese Historiography and Historians (二十世紀史學與史學家). Taipei: Tonson Publications, 2021.

Xingzai Shuo Zhongguo 幸仔說中國 (Lucky Talk China). "After a Full Year of Making a Scene, When Will Fang Fang Get What is Coming to Her? Today We Have an Answer!" ("Fang Fang naoteng le yi nian, shenme shihou shoushi ta? Jintian you daan!" 方方鬧騰了一年，什麼時候收拾她?今天有答案!) Uploaded to Youtube on February 2, 2021. https://www.youtube.com/watch?v=i I4NBPWR95g

Xingzai shuo Zhongguo's 幸仔說中國 (Lucky Talks China). "Three Days After Biden Assumes Office, the United States has Suddenly Realized there is a Serious Problem! Fang Fang has Terribly Deceived them! Life in China is Good!" ("Baideng shangtai 3 tian, Meiguo turan yishidao yige zhongyao wenti! Fang Fang ba tamen piancan le! Shenghuo zai Zhongguo zhen xingfu!" 拜登上台3天，美國突然意識到一個重要問題!方方把他們騙慘了!生活在中國真幸福!) Uploaded to Youtube on January 23, 2021. https://www.youtube.com/watch?v=6Mjljle795Q

Xinhua News Wuhan Frontline Reporting Team. *The Battle for Wuhan: Diaries of Journalists on the COVID-19 Frontline. (Wuhan zhanyi riji).* Beijing: Xinhua chubanshe, 2020.

Xu Xiaodong 徐曉東. Youtube video denouncing Lei Lei: https://www.youtube.com/watch?v=zc5f6dCsxa4

Yam Bear Six 地瓜熊老六. "American Diary 191: 2020 seems to be a big glorious year for FF; but actually it has been a shameless year of lament" ("Meiguo riji 191: 2020 maosi FF de fengguang danian, shize gengshi ta de wuchi ainian" 美國日記191:2020貌似FF的風光大年，實則更是她的無恥哀年) October, 5, 2020 on Weibo: https://weibo.com/ttarticle/p/show?id=2309404556812870353181#_0

Yan Geling 嚴歌苓 "Hide! Hide! Hide" (瞞!瞞!瞞!)Translated by Nicky Harman. Paper Republic website: https://paper-republic.org/pubs/read/hide-hide-hide/

Yan Lianke 閻連科. "What Happens After Coronavirus? On Community Memory and Repeating Our Own Mistakes" 2020 Literary Hub, March 11, 2020. https://lithub.com/yan-lianke-what-happens-after-coronavirus/

Yang, Guobin. "In China, Pandemic Diaries Unite, and Divide, a Nation" in Social Science Research Council, Items, Insights from the Social Sciences, September 24, 2020a. https://items.ssrc.org/covid-19-and-the-social-sciences/mediated-crisis/in-china-pandemic-diaries-unite-and-divide-a-nation/?fbclid=IwAR1HmfnaxGU2VLCxwhUc1lZ1pOhn7RDXdH2WLXrhKfLL6XR7lZQ6TNs0piQ

Yang, Guobin. "In China, Pandemic Diaries Unite, and Divide, a Nation" in Social Science Research Council, Items, Insights from the Social Sciences, September 24, 2020b. https://items.ssrc.org/covid-19-and-the-social-sciences/mediated-crisis/in-china-pandemic-diaries-unite-and-divide-a-nation/?fbclid=IwAR1HmfnaxGU2VLCxwhUc1lZ1pOhn7RDXdH2WLXrhKfLL6XR7lZQ6TNs0piQ

Yang, Guobin. *The Power of the Internet in China: Citizen Activism Online.* New York, Columbia University Press, 2009.

Yang, Guobin. "Performing Cyber-Nationalism in Twenty-First Century China: The Case of Diba Expedition" in Liu, Hailong ed. *From Cyber-Nationalism to Fandom Nationalism: The Case of Diba Expedition in China.* New York: Routledge, 2020c. Pgs. 1–12.

Yang, Guobin. *The Wuhan Lockdown.* New York: Columbia University Press: 2021

Jinquan Yu, Binghan Zheng and Lu Shao. "Who has the final say? English translation of online lockdown writing *Wuhan Diary*" in *Perspectives: Studies in Translation Theory and Practice.* Routledge. Published online May 26, 2021. https://doi.org/10.1080/0907676X.2021.1928251

Yu Nie 余涅. "Some Remarks on the Investigation into Hubei University Professor Liang Yanping" ("Tantan Hubei daxue diaocha Liang Yanping jiaoshou" 〈談

談湖北大學調查梁艷萍教授〉) on Red China (RedChinaCn.net) on April 28, 2020.   http://redchinacn.org/forum.php?mod=viewthread&tid=16793&ex tra=page%3D1

Zha Qiongfang. *Dr Zha's Diary of Fighting the COVID-19*. Shanghai: Shanghai Jiao Tong University Press, 2020.

Zhang Ling 張翎. *Panic on the Road: My Experience During the Coronavirus Outbreak* (*Yi lu huangkong: Wo de yicheng jishi* 一路惶恐:我的疫情記事). Taipei: China Times, 2020.

Zhang Sheng 張生. "Professor Michael Berry" ("Bai Ruiwen jiaoshou" 白睿文教授) originally posted to Weibo on April 16, 2020, reprinted on numerous websites, including: https://posts.careerengine.us/p/5ead539fff7e81298ce3071a

Zhang Yuanke 張元珂 (ed.). *Research Materials on Fang Fang* (*Fang Fang yanjiu ziliao* 方方研究資料). Nanchang: Baihuazhou Literature and Art Press, 2019.

Zhao Dongfang 趙東方. *Diary of the Battle Against the Virus at Leishenshan* (*Leishenshan zhanyi riji* 雷神山戰疫日記). Wuhan: Hubei People's Publishing House, 2020.

Zhao Keming 趙可銘. "*Soft Burial* is Vindictive Counterattack Against the Land Reform Movement" ("Ruanmai shi dui tugai de fangongdaosuan" 《軟埋》是對土改的反攻倒算) in Red Culture Online (Hongse wenhua wang紅色文化網), May 25, 2017. http://www.hswh.org.cn/wzzx/llyd/zz/2017-05-22/44243.html

Zhuang Pinghui. "The rise of the Little Pink: China's angry young digital warriors" South China Morning Post. May 26, 2017. https://www.scmp.com/news/china/society/article/2095458/rise-little-pink-chinas-young-angry-digital-warriors

Zhong, Raymond, Paul Mozur, Jeff Kao and Aaron Krolik. "No 'Negative' News: How China Censored the Coronavirus" New York Times, December 19, 2020. https://www.nytimes.com/2020/12/19/technology/china-coronavirus-censorship.html?smid=em-share

Žižek, Slavoj. *Pandemic!: COVID-19 Shakes the World*. New York: Polity Press, 2020.

Index[1]

---

[1] Note: Page numbers followed by 'n' refer to notes.

221

L

Lai Fu 來福, 57
Land Reform Movement, 22, 23, 53
Legal debates (surrounding Wuhan
   Diary), 173
Lei Lei 雷雷 (Wei Lei 魏雷), 110,
   112–114, 112n12
Leishenshan Hospital 雷神山醫院,
   122, 167
Les Misérables, 90
"A Lesson for Fang Fang" (Gei Fang
   Fang shang yi ke 給方方上一課),
   87–89, 88n2
"Let's Go Brandon," 114
"Literary Scum: Diss Fang Fang"
   (Wenzha 文渣), 106
Li Wenliang 李文亮, 16, 90, 92, 127,
   168, 175, 180, 197
Li Xueying 李雪穎, 121, 127, 175
Li Zehua 李澤華, 174
Liang Yanping 梁艷萍, 92–95,
   94n16, 97, 157
Liao Guangsheng 廖光生, 170
Liao Yiwu 廖亦武, 143
Lin Zhao 林昭, 28
Little Kitty's Diary: The Kitty with a
   Facemask (Xiaomao riji dai
   kouzhao de mao 小貓日記:戴口罩
   的貓), 124
Little Pinks (xiao fenhong 小粉紅), 67,
   97, 102, 104, 154, 161, 163, 208
Little Red Soldiers (hongse xiaobing
   紅色小兵), 161
Liu Binyan 劉賓雁, 28, 146n8
Liu Xiaobo 劉曉波, 28, 143
Liu Xinglong 劉醒龍, 142
Liu Yingzi 劉英姿, 198
Liu, Chang, 106
Liu Chuan-e 劉川鄂, 92–93
Liu, Eric, 72, 90, 165
Liu, Simu, 196

Liu, Yi-Ling, 108
Lockdown diaries (fengcheng riji 封城
   日記), 41, 116n1
Lockdown diary, 42, 49, 51, 143
The London Times, 71, 119
Los Angeles, 2, 3, 6, 79, 142,
   143, 192
The Los Angeles Times, 71, 192
Lu Han 鹿晗, 142
Lu, Pinyue 魯品越, 83
Lu Xun's 魯迅, 13–15, 52, 53, 98,
   109, 149, 182
Lu Yao Literary Prize, 23
Lucky Talks China (Xingzai shuo
   Zhongguo 幸仔說中國),
   149–151, 150n14, 150n15
Lung Yingtai's 龍應台, 182

M

Ma Guoqiang 馬國強, 198
"A Madman's Diary" (Kuangren riji
   狂人日記), 14, 15, 52, 98, 182
Make America Great Again, 191
Mao Zedong 毛澤東, 22–27, 53, 85,
   97, 99, 100, 102, 148, 160,
   161, 170
Masks, see Facemasks
Mayo, Katherine, 11
McCarthy, Joe, 54
"Medicine" ("Yao" 藥), 98
The Mermaid (Meirenyu 美人鱼), 109
Militarization of the virus
   narrative, 125n12
Ministry of Propaganda, 73, 187
Minority Report, 170
MIT, 189
Mo Yan 莫言, 26, 31
Mother India, 11
Mulan, 192
Mullinax, Tzu-I Chuang 莊祖宜, 157

Printed in Dunstable, United Kingdom